Coping with Illness Digitally

Coping with Illness Digitally

Stephen A. Rains

The MIT Press
Cambridge, Massachusetts
London, England

This book was set in ITC Stone Sans Std and ITC Stone Serif Std by Toppan Best-set Premedia Limited. Printed and bound in the United States of America.

Library of Congress Cataloging-in-Publication Data

Names: Rains, Stephen A., author.
Title: Coping with illness digitally / Stephen A. Rains.
Description: Cambridge, MA : The MIT Press, [2018] | Includes bibliographical
   references and index.
Identifiers: LCCN 2017057485 | ISBN 9780262038287 (hardcover : alk. paper)
Subjects: LCSH: Communication in medicine. | Social media in medicine. |
   Patients--Social networks. | Online social networks.
Classification: LCC R118 .R24 2018 | DDC 610.285--dc23 LC record available at
https://lccn.loc.gov/2017057485

10 9 8 7 6 5 4 3 2 1

This book is dedicated to Katie Kennealy and Carol Young for their indomitable spirits in battling cancer.

Contents

Contents

Acknowledgments

I am grateful to the many people who helped make this book possible. Gita Manaktala, Jesus Hernandez, and the team at MIT Press are a central reason that this book appears in print. Beyond giving me the opportunity to publish my work, they provided valuable feedback and shepherded me through the publication process. I greatly appreciate their assistance. I am also indebted to the five anonymous reviewers who evaluated my proposal and complete manuscript. The issues they identified helped me to produce what I believe to be a stronger and more coherent book.

I am grateful to my colleagues who were a valuable resource throughout this project. I appreciate the generosity of Kory Floyd, Jake Harwood, Craig Scott, and Chris Segrin in sharing drafts of their previous proposals, offering insights about the book-publishing process, and encouraging me to undertake this endeavor. Chris and Craig were also incredibly generous with their time in reviewing the model presented in the final chapter. They provided thoughtful feedback that helped me to substantially improve and expand the model.

I am grateful to my current and former students with whom I collaborated on a number of studies reviewed in this book. Chelsie Akers, Steven Brunner, Dave Keating, Corey Pavlich, Erin Ruppel, Bobby Tokunaga, and Eric Tsetsi have played an instrumental role in helping me study digital coping. I am thankful for their efforts to advance our work and their enthusiasm in pursuing these endeavors.

Finally, I am grateful to my wife, Jamie Kennealy, and son, Will Rains, for their endless support. They endured countless dinners hearing about the challenges involved in writing this book and yet continued to inquire about my progress. I am incredibly thankful for their patience and encouragement.

1 Introduction

Serious illness can have a profound impact on virtually every aspect of one's life. Physical symptoms may limit one's mobility and competence to perform basic tasks. Concerns for the future or thoughts about mortality can tax one's psychological well-being. The demands that one's illness places on friends and family who serve as caregivers can strain one's most important relationships. The technical aspects of one's condition and need to navigate a potentially complicated medical system can be significant sources of frustration. Missed work, deductibles, and co-pays can create substantial financial burden. Even one's professional aspirations and career trajectory may be threatened by illness.

Although the medical dimensions of illness tend to receive much of the attention, researchers have increasingly begun to consider its psychological and social consequences. Illness has been examined in terms of the disruption it causes to the structure of everyday life (Bury, 1982). Others have evaluated the ways in which people make sense of serious illness (Kleinman, 1988; Sontag, 1977). These works share an assumption that coping with illness extends well beyond remedying the malfunction of one's body. Illness is a complex and ever-changing set of experiences. Coping with it involves an equally sophisticated set of activities.

The past quarter century has been marked by the widespread diffusion of communication technologies largely made possible by personal computers and the Internet. Surveys conducted by researchers at the Pew Internet and American Life Project (PIALP) and National Cancer Institute (NCI) indicate that Internet use among adult Americans has stabilized at approximately 80 percent. From e-mail and instant messaging to contemporary forms of social media such as social network sites (SNSs) and blogs, these technologies offer novel opportunities for people to interact and share their lives with others. It is perhaps not surprising that these technologies would be used for health-related purposes. Indeed, communication technologies may be used to acquire health information, find and evaluate a health care provider, learn about others' experiences with a health condition, participate in peer support communities, as well as numerous other activities.

The central premise of this book is that fully understanding the process of coping with illness in contemporary society requires considering the role of communication technologies. Its purpose is to evaluate the promise and peril of digital coping—or the use of communication technologies in responding to illness. Existing empirical research is synthesized to gain insights about how and with what effects patients use communication technologies, particularly social media, as a coping resource. The book culminates in a comprehensive model of digital coping. Taken as a whole, this book offers an in-depth look at what it means to cope with illness digitally.

This introductory chapter proceeds with an overview of health-related Internet use in contemporary society and the potential role of communication technologies as a coping resource. Key concepts are then defined and the remaining chapters previewed. Readers should leave this chapter with a clear understanding of what can be learned from this book.

Coping with Illness and the Role of Communication Technologies

Health-related uses of communication technologies have a fairly long history in the United States. During the Civil War, the telegraph provided a means to share information about casualties and medical supplies (Zundel, 1996). Shortly after its invention in the late 1800s, the telephone was employed by patients and health providers (Spielberg, 1998). Patients used the telephone to contact providers in the case of emergencies, and providers relied on it to communicate with pharmacies. During the late 1950s, efforts at understanding the potential of telemedicine began in earnest (Bashshur & Shannon, 2009). Systematic attempts were made to evaluate the utility of audio and video technologies for delivering health care.

A turning point in the evolution of health-related communication technology use occurred during the start of the twentieth century. The estimated 18.6 percent of U.S. households that had Internet access during 1997 ballooned to more than 60 percent during 2003 (National Telecommunication and Information Agency, 2004). As of 2015, an estimated 84 percent of all adult Americans used the Internet—a number that has remained fairly consistent during the previous five years (Perrin & Duggan, 2015). The rapid and widespread diffusion of personal computers and the Internet created an infrastructure for many of the most popular contemporary communication technologies. In addition to "older" technologies such as e-mail and instant messaging, SNSs, blogs, microblogs, and other forms of social media have all been adopted for health-related uses.

Researchers working at the PIALP and NCI have conducted a series of surveys over the past decade to investigate health-related uses of the Internet and personal computers. In one of the earliest surveys conducted during 2000, 55 percent of Internet users were estimated to have gone online in search of health information (Rainie & Fox, 2000). More than 90 percent of those information seekers reported finding useful health information online. Several other health-related online activities were also identified. One in ten information seekers, for example, communicated with a doctor or purchased medicine/vitamins online. Since that time, researchers have identified a myriad of other health-related Internet uses. Table 1.1 summarizes the results from PIALP and NCI surveys conducted between 2011 and 2015.

As illustrated in table 1.1, a primary function of the Internet continues to be as a health information resource. Three-quarters of all Internet users have searched for health information online, and more than one-third have looked for information about a health care provider. It is noteworthy that, although both of these types of information are available, they tend to be much more difficult to acquire offline. Beyond finding information, health-related Internet use serves distinctly social purposes. Almost one-third of all Internet users have e-mailed their health care provider or their provider's office. In addition to interacting with health professionals, the Internet is being used to connect with and learn about other members of the lay public who are concerned with a particular health issue. Such uses range from viewing the insights and experiences of people coping with a particular condition to consulting other patients' evaluations of a health provider.

Although health-related Internet use appears to be fairly widespread, evidence indicates that it is more prevalent among some demographic groups than others. Researchers have analyzed survey data from the NCI

Table 1.1
Health-Focused Internet Use Identified in PIALP and NCI Surveys (2011–2015)

Health-related online activities performed by U.S. adults	Percent of Internet users who have performed this activity
Searched for health information for oneself[1]	76
Looked for a health care provider[1]	42
Used e-mail to communicate with a doctor or doctor's office[2]	30
Read or watched someone else's experiences with a health issue[3]	26
Visited a SNS to read or share about medical issues[2]	23
Purchased medicine or vitamins[2]	20
Consulted reviews or rakings of health providers[3]	17
Tried to find others who share the same health concerns[3]	16
Posted a health-related review or ranking[3]	7
Participated in a health-focused support community[1]	5
Authored a health-focused blog[4]	3

[1]National Cancer Institute (2015).
[2]National Cancer Institute (2013).
[3]Pew Internet and American Life Project (2012).
[4]National Cancer Institute (2011).

to identify who engages in activities such as seeking medical information, looking for a health care provider, e-mailing a health care provider, tracking diet and exercise activity online, participating in a health-related online support community or SNS, or blogging about health (Kontos, Blake, Chou, & Prestin, 2014; Prestin, Vieux, & Chou, 2015). Adults who were younger, more educated, and female tended to be more likely to use communication technologies for such health purposes. There were, however, exceptions to these trends. People with lower levels of education, for example, tended to be more likely to use SNSs and online support communities.

Researchers have also begun to consider broader trends in people's use of communication technologies as a coping resource. Ziebland and Wyke (2012) proposed several different pathways through which social media are used by patients. One important use involves giving and receiving information. Through hearing about the experiences of others facing a similar health concern, one may learn strategies for managing symptoms, tips for dealing with doctors, and expectations for the condition's trajectory. Social media also offers opportunities to share difficulties and receive emotional support. Other people who are facing or have faced similar circumstances are in a unique position to provide empathy. A third use of social media involves the opportunity to create and maintain relationships with others facing the same condition. Such relationships can play a valuable role in allowing people experiencing illness to acclimate to their role and identity as a patient.

In summary, communication technologies appear to have potentially significant implications for health and illness. It is clear that the Internet is being used for a variety of health-related purposes. Although researchers are beginning to consider the consequences of such uses, a comprehensive exploration of this topic is desperately needed. An in-depth analysis of digital coping is presented in this book. It will contribute substantive insights about how people cope with illness and the broader implications of communication technologies in contemporary society.

Overview of the Book

Having identified the potential significance of communication technologies in coping with illness, it is important to provide readers with a preview of this book. In the following sections, the central objectives pursued in the book are identified, key assumptions are explained, and important terms are defined. A summary of the remaining chapters is then offered. Readers should leave this section with clear expectations about what they can and cannot expect to learn from this book.

Objectives

The goal of this book is to advance our understanding of how, why, and with what effects communication technologies are being used in coping with illness. Two more specific objectives are pursued in an effort to achieve this end. The first involves synthesizing existing research examining the implications of communication technologies—particularly social media—among patients. Although a sizeable body of scholarship has accumulated, these works remain disconnected. Existing research has been conducted by scholars working across a diverse range of disciplines from the social sciences to computer science and medicine. Researchers have focused on a myriad of technologies, health conditions, and coping activities. In this book, I attempt to summarize what is and is not known about the use and consequences of communication technologies among patients. My hope is that this effort will offer scholars, students, healthcare professionals, and the general public insights about the implications of communication technologies as a coping resource.

A second objective pursued in this book is the development of a model explicating the process of digital coping. The purpose of the model is to identify and summarize the key functions of communication technologies during the coping process. The model is not limited to any specific illness or communication technology. It is applicable to a range of health conditions and communication technologies—including those technologies that might be developed in the future. The model is intended to be useful to a wide audience. For students and health care professionals, the model illustrates when and why communication technologies may be consequential. For scholars, the model offers a framework to understand the central elements and functions of digital coping along with an agenda for future research.

In discussing the objectives of this book, it is also useful to consider those topics that will not be addressed. This book is neither intended nor sufficient as a formal medical text on the treatment of any one condition or illness more generally. Although some of the ideas examined may have implications for treatment, no specific medical treatments are discussed or advocated. Moreover, the book does not focus on any one illness or health condition. It is intended to be sufficiently general to apply to a wide range of illnesses and health conditions. This book does not address technical issues related to computer programming or design. Programmers and designers may glean insights from this text about how communication technologies are used by patients, but technical topics related to computer science will not be discussed. Finally, this book does not consider ethical or legal issues related to communication technologies or health. As with the preceding topics, legal and ethical scholars might benefit from reading this book, but specific issues related to these two subjects are not explicitly examined.

Key Assumptions

Two basic assumptions ground this book and shape its focus and scope. The first assumption, which stems from the biopsychosocial approach to health and illness (Engel, 1977; Suls & Rothman, 2004), is that one's social world plays a critical role in health. Illness and responses to illness are shaped in part by social processes involving one's connections and interactions with other humans. The research examined in this book reflects this assumption. The vast majority of primary studies considered in the following chapters explore how, why, and with what effects people experiencing illness use communication technologies for social purposes. Human–computer interaction is not widely considered in this text. Similarly, nonsocial uses of technologies, such as tracking technologies designed to monitor one's diet or fitness, receive little attention. Although these topics are certainly worthy of study, they exceed the scope of the present project. This book emphasizes the social implications of communication technologies among people coping with illness.

A second assumption involves the approach adopted in this book for thinking about communication technologies. The implications of communication technologies are assumed to be contingent on the context in which they are used. Technologies are investigated as a means for engaging in coping activities. This assumption has consequences for the form and structure of this book. As opposed to focusing on single technologies such as search engines or online communities in isolation, the book is organized around several distinct classes of coping activities, and the affordances that transcend individual technologies are privileged. Although research on specific technologies will be considered, the individual technologies are examined as exemplars of broader affordances used to engage in coping activities. This book focuses on exploring how affordances of technologies are used—and with what effects—in the process of coping with illness.

Some readers might understandably question the decision to not focus on or privilege individual communication technologies. Indeed, one might imagine a book with separate chapters dedicated to online communities, SNSs, personal monitoring devices, mobile phone applications, and other technologies. Such an approach was not adopted in this project for two reasons. First, given the fairly rapid development and diffusion of new technologies like various forms of social media in recent years, any attempt to consolidate research on individual technologies is destined to become rapidly dated as technologies evolve or become obsolete and new(er) communication technologies emerge. Second, in privileging individual technologies, we risk losing sight of the connections among and across technologies. Focusing on single technologies in isolation can make it difficult to see the broader implications of communication technology in coping with illness.

The approach to studying communication technologies adopted in this text also has some important advantages. One such advantage involves the potential for the ideas in this text to remain relevant over an extended period of time. Although the potential to rapidly become obsolete is present in virtually any academic endeavor involving the study of communication technologies, the approach adopted in this text reduces this threat. Through investigating technology use in the context of a broader coping activity and considering those affordances that transcend individual technologies, it will be possible to identify some essential dimensions of health-related technology use. Although individual technologies for seeking social support or health information may come and go, the underlying affordances and coping behaviors should persist. Another advantage of the approach adopted in this book involves its potential contribution to our understanding of communication technologies. As previously noted, considering affordances that pervade different technologies helps us gain greater insights about the consequences of communication technology more broadly in contemporary society. Finally, the approach adopted in this text offers considerable potential for advancing our knowledge about how people cope with illness. Through highlighting coping activities, we learn about the ways in which people respond to illness in a contemporary society marked by fairly widespread use of communication technologies.

Definitions for Important Terms

In addition to discussing the objectives for this book, several key terms must be defined. *Illness* is conceptualized broadly as involving an individual's "experiences of disvalued changes in states of being and in social function" (Eisenberg, 1977, p. 11). It is distinguished from the notion of *disease*, which focuses on defects in the functioning of one's body. Whereas disease has medical connotations involving specific mental or physical systems, illness is a more general construct encompassing one's beliefs, actions, and experiences related to one's state of being (Kleinman, 1988).

The term *patient* is used throughout the book to identify people experiencing illness. As with the notion of illness, the construct patient is defined broadly. One need not receive a formal diagnosis from a medical doctor to be considered a patient. Moreover, no one specific health condition is privileged. Research related to people coping with conditions that are chronic or acute, mental or physical, terminal or nonterminal are all addressed. Of central importance in this book is how people experience and respond to these conditions. Although much of the research reviewed will focus on people who are currently coping with illness, some will involve those who were previously ill, are concerned about becoming ill, or serve as caregivers.

The term *coping* is similarly conceptualized broadly to include one's efforts to respond to illness. Following Lazarus (1993), coping is defined as involving "ongoing cognitive and behavioral efforts to manage specific external and/or internal demands that are appraised as taxing or exceeding the resources of the person" (p. 237). Coping is an ongoing and evolving process. It is made up of discrete activities that may ebb, flow, and change over time. Although the term coping tends to have positive connotations, it will not be assumed to necessarily result in objectively beneficial outcomes. Several instances throughout the book will be identified where coping has negative outcomes or is otherwise maladaptive.

Communication technologies are conceptualized as including Internet-based technologies that function to connect people and allow for human interaction. Much of the research reviewed in this book will focus on social media. Although definitions of social media vary (e.g., Kaplan & Haenlein, 2010; Leonardi, Huysman, & Steinfield, 2013), most highlight the importance of user-generated content. Online communities are perhaps the earliest form of social media and are composed of and sustained by the messages contributed by individual members. More contemporary forms include SNSs, blogs, microblogs, video-sharing sites, photo-sharing sites, social bookmarking sites, and other technologies. Older communication technologies that make possible interaction between two or more people, such as e-mail and instant messaging, will also be considered. The implications of mobile phones or other health technologies, however, are beyond the scope of this book and will not be addressed in any depth.

Although research on a range of specific technologies such as blogs, SNSs, and online communities will be discussed, the book tends to focus on those uses and effects that transcend individual technologies. Throughout each of the following chapters, the affordances of communication technologies that are unique to each context will be considered. An affordance involves the way a technology is perceived and used (Gibson, 1977; Markus & Silver, 2008; Norman, 1999). A distinction can be drawn between affordances and features. Whereas features focus on the technical dimensions of a technology such as the ability to communicate using written language, affordances concern how such features are interpreted and acted on by users. The potential to communicate using writing language may lend itself to an affordance of documentation, whereby patients facing a terminal illness use communication technologies to leave a record of their life history for their friends and family.

Organizational Structure

This book is organized around a series of chapters that align with specific challenges raised by illness. Chapter 2 will consider the implications of communication technologies for patients' social connections. The motivations and outcomes related to making connections online will be discussed along with the properties of patients' online health networks. Chapters 3 and 4 explore the use of communication technologies to share illness experiences and marshal social support resources. These chapters will consider the consequences of making health disclosures and exchanging support online. Chapter 5 will discuss health information seeking online and, in particular, how communication technologies are used to address the bevy of questions that accompany illness. Chapter 6 explores the implications of communication technologies for patients and health providers. A central focus of this chapter will be on understanding how and why the Internet has impacted patient–provider relations. Chapter 7 considers the role of communication technologies at the end of life and in bereavement. In the final chapter of the book, an original model of digital coping is presented. The model builds on issues discussed in the previous chapters in an effort to summarize the potential role and consequences of communication technologies in coping with illness.

Chapters 2 through 7 have the same basic structure. They begin with a brief overview of important ideas about the broader topic that defines the chapter. The bulk of each chapter then focuses on synthesizing existing research regarding the implications of communication technologies in that particular context. A section is also included in which the unique affordances of communication technologies are considered. These affordances are central to the model developed in final chapter. Chapters 2 through 7 conclude with a summary of issues warranting greater attention.

Conclusion

Given the pervasive nature of communication technologies in the everyday life of many people around the world, it is perhaps not surprising that they might be used for coping with illness. Indeed, the central premise of this book is that communication technologies have important implications for coping efforts. This chapter serves as a foundation for the remainder of the book. Background information about health-related technology use was provided, key terms used in the book were defined, and an overview was outlined. The following chapters will focus on exploring the implications of communication technologies in specific contexts and culminate in an original model of digital coping.

2 Making and Reinforcing Connections

Serious illness can be isolating (Royer, 1998). The unique experiences that define illness can set patients apart from others. Despite their best intentions, friends and family may have difficulty fully understanding the nuances or magnitude of a patient's circumstances. In some instances, they may even withdraw or otherwise become distant. Illness can also make it challenging for patients to maintain contact with others. Beyond any mobility impairments, illness may make it hard to perform routine activities that involve social interaction. The inability to continue working, for example, may serve to substantially reduce one's contact with others. Illness can leave patients detached from their social network.

The thesis of this chapter is that communication technologies have important implications for forming and maintaining connections among people experiencing illness. The chapter begins with background information about the role of social relationships in health. Motivations for and outcomes of pursuing social connections online are next considered. The properties of patients' social networks online are then evaluated. The chapter concludes with a discussion of issues warranting additional attention in scholarship on communication technologies, social relationships, and illness.

Illness and Social Connection

Background on Social Relationships and Health
Social relationships play an important role in health and well-being. In a review of almost 150 studies examining the mortality rates of more than 300,000 people, researchers found that individuals with stronger social relationships had a 50 percent greater likelihood of survival (Holt-Lunstad,

Smith, & Layton, 2010). Compared to people with poorer relationships, people with more robust relationships were generally less likely to die from a wide range of causes. This basic finding has been observed in numerous other studies (House, Landis, & Umberson, 1988; Uchino, 2009). Having meaningful social relationships can serve a variety of pro-health functions.

The link between one's social connections and health has been the focus of research on social integration (Berkman & Glass, 2000; Brissette, Cohen, & Seeman, 2000; Thoits, 2011). As an umbrella term referring to several phenomena, social integration generally involves the implications of participating in a social network. Although several approaches have been advanced for understanding social integration (Cohen & Wills, 1985; Thoits, 2011; Wills & Ainette, 2012), one of the most comprehensive was presented by Berkman and Glass (2000). They outlined a broad process to explain how social structure, social networks, and psychosocial mechanisms contribute to health through specific pathways. Most relevant to this chapter, properties of social networks create opportunities for exposure to mechanisms such as social support, social influence, social engagement, and access to resources. These mechanisms impact specific behavioral pathways (e.g., exercise), psychological pathways (e.g., self-efficacy), or physiological pathways (e.g., allostatic load) that directly influence health and well-being.

Social network analysis has been one valuable approach for understanding the health-related implications of social relationships (Smith & Christakis, 2008). As a theoretical perspective and method, social network analysis makes it possible to examine human behavior within networks of people and gain insights about how networks serve to influence the behavior of individual members (Berkman & Glass, 2000; Rosenquist, 2011). Individuals are situated within broader networks of ties or relations (e.g., family, friends, coworkers, etc.) who themselves are connected to networks of ties. These networks can directly or indirectly impact individual members' health. Social network analysis also offers insights into the spread of health perceptions, behaviors, and outcomes within a community.

Affordances of Communication Technologies for Making and Reinforcing Connections

Having discussed the general link between social relationships and health as well as the importance of social networks, it is necessary to consider affordances of communication technologies that are particularly important for making and reinforcing connections. Communication technologies such as social network sites (SNSs), blogs, online communities, e-mail, and others can be distinguished based on the relative presence or absence of several different affordances. Four that are particularly relevant in this context include visibility, availability, control, and reach. Each of these affordances is summarized in table 2.1.

Visibility involves the potential to make one's self known to others or to observe others' behavior. Communication technologies create opportunities for patients to make others aware of their issue or to witness others' coping behaviors. This could take the form of creating a blog to share one's illness experiences with friends and extended family members or reading a contribution to an online community authored by another patient. Visibility may be particularly useful in attempting to overcome the sense of isolation that can accompany illness. Patients can feel as if they are alone in confronting their circumstances (Hinton, Kurinczuk, & Ziebland, 2010; Holbrey & Colson, 2013; Yli-Uotila, Rantanen, & Suominen, 2014). The visibility provided by online communities, blogs, SNSs, and other technologies offers the potential to ameliorate isolation by identifying other patients or making friends and family aware of one's concerns.

Availability is a second affordance involving the accessibility of others. Communication technologies vary in the degree and ways in which they make it possible to overcome time and space constraints that may serve to limit patients' potential to connect with others. Asynchronous technologies like such as online communities, e-mail, and blogs allow people to communicate without being co-present. Unlike a telephone conversation, messages can be sent and received at different times. This may be critical

Table 2.1
Affordances of Communication Technologies for Social Connection

Affordance	Definition
Visibility	Potential to make one's self known to others or observe others' behavior.
Availability	Potential to overcome time and space constraints in connecting with others.
Control	Potential to manage aspects of human interaction.
Reach	Potential to contact specific individuals, groups, or communities.

for patients to maintain connections with friends or caregivers who face restrictions on when they may interact (Liu, Inkpen, & Pratt, 2015). Availability can also involve the potential to overcome geographic distance. One need not be in the same physical space as one's interaction partner. This can be particularly important for patients with restricted mobility (Markle, Attell, & Treiber, 2015; Rodriquez, 2013). Patients can maintain existing connections and form new ones without the need to leave home.

Control is a third affordance that concerns the potential to manage interactions. Communication technologies can offer various mechanisms for controlling interactions. The text-based nature of technologies such as online communities and blogs makes is possible for patients to discuss their thoughts and feelings outside of the direct gaze of others. Similarly, the asynchronous nature of these technologies gives patients the potential to revise their messages prior to sharing. Particularly given the intimate nature of illness, patients may be wary of sharing their thoughts and experiences (Yeshua-Katz & Martins, 2013). Doing so could involve talking about things that are embarrassing or otherwise might invite unwanted scrutiny. The ability to control some aspects of interaction creates opportunities for patients to feel more comfortable and perhaps even be more effective in forming and maintaining social connections.

Reach is the final affordance relevant to making connections, involving the potential to contact specific others. In the case of making connections, reach tends to concern the potential for contacting individuals, groups, or communities who share key similarities. SNSs, online communities, blogs, and other technologies offer the potential to find and interact with a potentially sizeable number of peers facing the same or a similar health issue. Their shared experiences can make peers a valuable asset for advice and empathy (Holbrey & Colson, 2013). More broadly, reach may also involve the opportunity to locate and participate in a community. The sense of inclusion, shared identity, and validation that accompany community membership can be an important coping resource (Dickins, Browning, Feldman, & Thomas, 2016).

Patients' Online Connections

Given the important role of social relationships in health and well-being (House et al., 1988; Uchino, 2009), it is perhaps not surprising that communication technologies would be used by patients to connect with others. A survey conducted by researchers at the Pew Internet and American Life Project during 2010 showed that 13 percent of adult Americans sought information, care, or support online from friends or family members the last time they had a health issue (Fox, 2011). During 2012, 16 percent of Internet users were estimated to have gone online specifically to locate others facing similar health concerns (Fox & Duggan, 2013). Notably, these surveys focused on U.S. adults in general and likely underestimate patients' use of communication technologies to connect with others. The volume of patients seeking connection online raises questions about the reasons that patients venture online and how doing so impacts their coping efforts. The most salient motivations and outcomes of pursuing social connections online will be considered in the following sections. They are summarized in table 2.2.

Motivations for Pursuing Social Connection Online

Four primary motivations appear to be driving patients to connect with others online. First, patients can be motivated by a desire to overcome feelings of isolation. Illness tends to involve an uncommon set of experiences that can serve to disconnect one from others. Members of an online community dedicated to infertility reported feeling like they did not fit in their existing social groups (Hinton et al., 2010). Members of breast cancer communities described entering a new world divorced from their existing social relationships (Høybye, Johansen, & Tjørnhøj-Thomsen, 2005). Feelings of isolation extended to perceptions of social exclusion. Bloggers writing about their experiences with obesity reported feeling disregarded and dismissed by society due to their condition (Dickins et al., 2016). Members of an online community dedicated to early onset Alzheimer's disease

Table 2.2
Key Motivations and Outcomes of Using Technologies for Social Connection

Motivations	Outcomes
• Overcoming isolation	• Membership in a community
• Identifying others with similar experiences	• Information acquisition
• Reinforcing existing relationships	• Normalization
• Offsetting deficits in existing relationships	• Relief from distress
	• Increased distress

experienced physical isolation after being forced to retire early from work and cease driving (Rodriquez, 2013).

The results of survey research have been less consistent but generally show a relationship between social isolation and patients' efforts to connect with others online. In a study of people experiencing negative life events, including illness, loneliness was positively associated with online coping efforts but not offline coping (van Ingen & Wright, 2016). People who were lonelier were more likely to report coping online. In another study, use of the discussion board and photo- and video-sharing applications in an online community were positively associated with the motivation to meet others (J. E. Chung, 2014). Other researchers, however, found no significant relationships between the frequency or intensity of social media use and loneliness among people with serious mental illness (Brusilovskiy, Townley, Snethen, & Salzer, 2016). Although not entirely uniform, the results from qualitative and quantitative research tend to indicate that patients are motivated to use communication technologies to overcome social isolation.

A second motivation for using communication technologies to connect with others concerns gaining access to peers who have similar illness experiences. People with comparable health conditions are in a unique position to understand one another's experiences (Thoits, 2011). Because they have gone through related physical, psychological, and social challenges, other patients can be a particularly valuable resource for information and empathy. Patients in several studies reported feeling that members of their online community were distinctly prepared to understand their health experiences (Colvin, Chenoeth, Bold, & Harding, 2004; Hadert & Rodham, 2008; Holbrey & Colson, 2013; Rodriquez, 2013). The motivation to communicate with similar others extends to participation in health-focused communities in the virtual world Second Life (Green-Hamann, Campbell Eichhorn, & Sherblom, 2011). This motivation has also been linked with maladaptive health behaviors. Pro-anorexia bloggers who embraced and promoted disordered eating reported that an important reason for maintaining their blog was to find others who could understand their experiences (Yeshua-Katz & Martins, 2013).

A third motivation for using communication technologies to connect with others involves reinforcing existing relationships. Patients may use communication technologies to increase their connections with family and friends. Blogs, in particular, appear to be a valuable tool for maintaining such relationships. A single blog post can update a broad swath of people about a patient's status or any new developments. Cancer patients reported using blogs to efficiently share their experiences with family and friends (McCosker & Darcy, 2013). In another study, blogging frequency was associated with new mothers' sense of social connection (McDaniel, Coyne, & Holmes, 2012). Mothers who blogged more frequently also reported feeling more connected with their existing friends and family members.

In addition to blogs, a wide range of technologies may be used to reinforce existing connections. In one study, use of the discussion board, photo and video sharing, and blog features of an online community were positively associated with patients' desire to maintain existing offline relationships (Chung, 2014). Patients who were motivated to reinforce their existing connections with friends and family members were more likely to use these technologies. Various technologies were used by children coping with a chronic health condition to keep in touch with their existing friends (Liu et al., 2015). Despite missing school or other events, texting and SNSs allowed them to continue their friendships. Yet other research conducted with the family members of a patient experiencing chronic illness suggests that some technologies may be better than others (Pang, Neustaedter, Riecke, Oduor, & Hillman, 2013). The telephone was perceived to be significantly more valuable than e-mail, videoconferencing, and SNSs for expressing emotion, maintaining engagement, and providing opportunities for social support. The telephone was also associated with greater feelings of obligation than the other technologies.

The final motivation for using communication technologies to make social connections entails patients' desire to offset or overcome deficiencies in their existing relationships. Patients may be motivated to acquire information and empathy that is unavailable or insufficient from their existing friends and family members. Because illness tends to be incredibly complex, family and friends may—despite their best efforts—have difficulty understanding and empathizing with a patient's experiences. Members of an online community dedicated to infertility, for example, noted that their friends and family were unable to fully grasp the challenges of their condition and anxiety associated with treatment (Malik & Coulson, 2008). Members of breast cancer communities similarly reported losing connection with their social networks once they became ill (Høybye et al., 2005).

In some cases, patients may even withhold their illness from family and friends. Members of a pro-anorexia online community were unable to share their condition with their closest friends and family or had experienced relational problems due to sharing (Gavin, Rodham, & Poyer, 2008). People facing early onset Alzheimer's disease (Rodriquez, 2013) and arthritis (Hadert & Rodham, 2008) reported that family and friends denied the existence of their condition or believed that the condition was fabricated.

Survey research has documented a link between the quality of patients' offline relationships and motivation to use communication technologies for social connection. Among online community members, people who had less support available from family and friends participated in the community more frequently (Cummings, Sproull, & Kiesler, 2002; Kim et al., 2011). Although not health focused, individuals who reported the least support available offline spent the most time participating in massively multiplayer online games (Kaczmarek & Krazkowski, 2014). Other researchers have reported an association between satisfaction with off- and online relationships. Online community members who were dissatisfied with their offline support sources showed the greatest preference for support from the community (J. E. Chung, 2013). In another study, online community members were more satisfied with the support they received from the community than from their offline connections (K. B. Wright, 2000).

These findings should be considered in light of other research showing no association between the quality of patients' offline relationships and motivation to make connections online. One group of researchers found no link between support from family and friends and use of an online community among patients with a hysterectomy (Bunde, Suls, Martin, & Barnett, 2006). In another study, time spent in online support communities was not correlated with members' satisfaction with face-to-face support (Wright, 1999). Taken as a whole, however, the quality of patients' existing relationships with friends and family members appears to be an important motivation for using communication technologies to connect with others.

Outcomes of Pursuing Social Connection Online

Beyond those factors that motivate patients to use communication technologies for social connection, several trends exist in the outcomes of such connections for patients' coping efforts. Although many of the outcomes tend to be constructive or beneficial, deleterious outcomes have been observed routinely. The five most prevalent outcomes will be considered in the following paragraphs.

First, through connecting with others online, patients may gain membership in a community. The common health conditions faced by bloggers, SNS users, and online community members can be a uniting force. Shared experiences were central to the sense of community reported by patients in several studies (Haberstroh & Moyer, 2012; Høybye et al., 2005). Patients had a similar set of experiences that made them feel part of something larger than themselves. Members of online communities dedicated to polycystic ovary syndrome (Holbrey & Colson, 2013), cancers (Yli-Uotila et al., 2014), and intentional self-injury (Haberstroh & Moyer, 2012) were moved by the knowledge that others deal with similar issues. Storytelling was integral to the development of community in another study (Rodriquez, 2013). Sharing stories that others could relate to helped reinforce the common experiences that bonded patients.

Community may serve several functions. Bloggers writing about obesity noted that their community helped to foster a sense of inclusion and protection (Dickins et al., 2016). Relief from isolation was evident in the comments posted to a video-sharing website about patients' experiences with serious mental illness (Naslund, Grande, Aschbrenner, & Elwyn, 2014). In one instance, community helped participants maintain a sense of abnormality (Gavin et al., 2008). The notion that one is not normal was central to a pro-anorexia group and reinforced by members as something that distinguished the group from nonmembers. Although community tended to be most frequently observed in studies of blogs and online communities, it was also evident in virtual worlds. In one study, members reported feeling a greater sense of community in their health-focused Second Life groups than in other online groups in which they had participated (Green-Hamann et al., 2011).

A second outcome of using communication technologies to connect with others pertains to acquiring information. Patients intentionally solicited information or were otherwise exposed to health-related information from their online connections (Holbrey & Colson, 2013). Online community members, for example, routinely reported being exposed to information about their condition as a direct result of their participation (Malik & Coulson, 2008). Information acquired from online connections served a variety of functions. It was used by patients to better understand their health condition, particularly among patients who had been diagnosed recently (Malik & Coulson, 2008). Information also influenced patients' relationships with their health providers and decision making (Hadert & Rodham, 2008). In one study, information obtained from others online was critical when patients perceived the information offered by their health provider to be inadequate (Markle et al., 2015). Similarly, the comments made in response to videos posted online by people facing serious mental illness included information about evaluating health providers and treatments (Naslund et al., 2014).

A third outcome of connecting with others online concerns normalization. In its broadest sense, normalization involves helping people come to terms with their illness. One component of normalization includes making illness, which tends to be uncommon, seem ordinary. Being around others facing the same health condition led members of an online community (Hinton et al., 2010) and video-sharing website (Hinton et al., 2010) to feel like their beliefs and behaviors were not unusual. In recognizing that others had similar feelings and responses, members of several online communities felt reassured (Attard & Coulson, 2012; Malik & Coulson, 2008). Validation also plays an important role in normalization. Patients coping with arthritis reported that their online community served to corroborate the existence of their symptoms (Hadert & Rodham, 2008). Normalization extends to integrating illness into one's life. For children with chronic illness, communication technologies played an important role in creating a "new normal" for their lives (Liu et al., 2015). This included using technology to connect with peers who were ill and manage relationships with existing friends. Blogging similarly helped adults experiencing multiple serious illnesses to retire their occupational identity and construct a new one (Markle et al., 2015).

A fourth outcome concerns achieving relief from distress. Connecting with others online allows patients to manage negative emotions. In several studies, online communities and blogs were used by patients to work through their health-related anxieties (Hinton et al., 2010; Ressler, Bradshaw, Gualtieri, & Chui, 2012). Members of online communities dedicated to cancer (Yli-Uotila et al., 2014), self-injury (Haberstroh & Moyer, 2012), and arthritis (Hadert & Rodham, 2008) described their communities as a place to relieve stress or vent negativity. Blogs similarly offered a place to manage the disruption associated with experiencing cancer (McCosker & Darcy, 2013). Beyond the potential to share one's distress, there is evidence that witnessing others' coping efforts can be beneficial. Members of one online community reported that reading about how others had managed the challenges of their condition led them to feel more optimistic (Holbrey & Colson, 2013).

Quantitative research offers further evidence of benefits of connecting with others online for relieving distress. In panel studies examining changes over extended periods of time, members of a breast cancer online community experienced increased posttraumatic growth (Lieberman & Goldstein, 2006), and members of a depression online community reported decreased levels of depression (Houston, Cooper, & Ford, 2002). These findings are consistent with survey research showing correlations between assessments of the utility of one's support community and one's level of stress or perceived coping ability (Seçkin, 2013; K. B. Wright, 2000). Members who reported more positive community evaluations felt lower levels of stress and greater levels of coping ability.

Although the previous outcomes tended to be positive, increased stress is a final outcome associated with using communication technologies for social connection. Using communication technologies can be upsetting for patients in numerous ways. In several studies of health-focused online communities, patients reported that reading about others' challenges and problems increased their own anxiety (Hadert & Rodham, 2008; Holbrey & Colson, 2013; Malik & Coulson, 2008). In addition to worrying about the negative things that could happen, hearing about others' difficulties was dispiriting. Making comparisons with other patients was a related source of distress (Malik & Coulson, 2008). Seeing others go through similar treatments and improve was upsetting for patients who had not experienced equivalent benefits. Participating in online communities led some members to become overly focused on their condition (Holbrey & Colson, 2013; Yli-Uotila et al., 2014). Bloggers coping with anorexia even reported that blogging had the potential to exacerbate their disordered eating behavior (Yeshua-Katz & Martins, 2013).

Distress can also stem from negative interactions with others online. In one study, receiving undesirable feedback from other community members led to anxiety among some patients (Yli-Uotila et al., 2014). The departure of community members who dropped out or failed to return was a challenge in another study (Attard & Coulson, 2012). It represented the loss of a confidant and was upsetting for some members. Among adults with autism, trouble maintaining computer-mediated relationships was challenging and, in some cases, even led to social rejection (Burke, Kraut, & Williams, 2010). Negative interactions were also linked to technological limitations such as the lack of social cues (Colvin et al., 2004) and the potential for a significant delay between when one requests and receives support (Haberstroh & Moyer, 2012).

To summarize, communication technologies can be valuable resources for patients to connect with others. The most prominent motivations for seeking connection stem from responding to the unique circumstances created by illness. The isolation associated with illness and desire to interact with others who have had similar experiences are important factors contributing to the use of communication technologies specifically to interact with previously unknown others. Yet technology use also may be motivated by a desire to reinforce existing relationships with friends and family. The outcomes of connecting with others largely involve the benefits of interacting with people facing similar health circumstances. Connecting with others allows patients to feel a sense of community, normalize their illness experiences, and acquire information. The outcomes of connecting, however, are not all positive. Connecting with others can be a source of significant distress for some patients in several different ways.

Networks of Connections Online

In addition to specific motivations and outcomes, it is important to consider broader trends in the implications of making connections online. Examining the networks formed online by patients offers valuable opportunities to gain insights into the ways in which communication technologies are being used as a coping resource. To this end, aggregate participation patterns in online patient groups will be discussed, followed by the structure and dynamics of online patient networks. Although the majority of this section involves online health communities, a diverse range of communication technologies will be represented.

Online Community Participation Patterns

Participation in health-focused online communities tends to follow a predictable pattern. A power law involves an exponential relationship between two variables (Himelboim, 2008; van Mierlo, Hyatt, & Ching, 2015). One power law that has been applied to explain participation in online health contexts is the 1 percent rule or the 90-9-1 principle (Carron-Arthur et al., 2016; van Mierlo, 2014). It predicts that a small proportion of members are responsible for an overwhelming majority of the participation in online communities (Carron-Arthur et al., 2016; van Mierlo, 2014). Only 1 percent of members are proposed to create the vast majority of content, whereas 9 percent contribute a modest amount and 90 percent contribute little to no content.

Evidence generally consistent with the 1 percent rule has been found in several studies. In an analysis of four different health communities and more than 60,000 people, a researcher identified three distinct groups that corresponded with the 1 percent rule (van Mierlo, 2014). Although super-users composed just 1 percent of all community members, they accounted for 74 percent of the posts made across the four communities. Contributors consisted of 9 percent of all community members and accounted for 24 percent of the content (i.e., posts made to the community). Lurkers made up the remaining 90 percent of members and contributed only 1 percent of the more than 500,000 posts made to the communities. In other research, an analysis of participation in a smoking cessation community over a 10-year period showed that the top 1 percent of users were responsible for 44 percent of the content, the next 9 percent were responsible for 44 percent, and the remaining 90 percent were responsible for 11 percent (Stearns, Nambiar, Nikolaev, Semenov, & McIntosh, 2014). Just 3 percent of users in another smoking cessation community contributed 69 percent of all the content (Healey, Hoek, & Edwards, 2014).

Beyond contributing content, evidence suggests that the 1 percent rule applies more broadly to participation and the number or nature of users' connections within an online health community (Ma, Chen, & Xiao, 2010). Researchers examining a smoking cessation community found that 90 percent of participants had established no connections in the community, 9 percent had a small number of ties, and 1 percent were responsible for most of the ties (Cobb, Graham, & Abrams, 2010). In a study examining several health communities on the website WebMD.com, researchers found that core network members who were densely connected represented fewer than 1 percent of all users (Introne, Semaan, & Goggins, 2016). Approximately 25 percent of users were periphery members, in that they engaged in at least one interaction with a core member, and the remaining 75 percent were deemed extra-periphery members because they played a small role in the community.

The nuances of patients' participation also appear to generally conform to the 1 percent rule. Online health communities are rife with people who visit a single time or are short-term members. Almost half of the participants in one community over a 10-year period were active on the site for only one day (Stearns et al., 2014). These people tended to participate in a single discussion, which for most tended to be the discussion thread they started. Fewer than 10 percent of users participated for more than a year. In an online community dedicated to psychosis, almost 75 percent of members contributed to only a single discussion thread (H.-J. Chang, 2009). Similarly, more than 60 percent of people who registered for a breast cancer community never returned (Wang, Kraut, & Levine, 2012).

The short-term nature of participation can also be observed in the lifespan of discussions. An analysis of contributions to the online support community hosted by the American Cancer Society showed that less than seven days passed between the first and final post in a thread for almost three-quarters of all discussions (Qiu et al., 2011). In a smoking cessation intervention, almost three-quarters of all initial posts to the discussion community came within three hours of when a given member registered (Selby, van Mierlo, Voci, Parent, & Cunningham, 2010). First posts that addressed a desire to quit smoking for health reasons were associated with less time between registering and posting.

Differences in Participation Patterns   Several factors can contribute to differences in participation among online health community members. A member's network or network position within the community is one important factor. People who are more central to the community tend to participate longer or more frequently. Core network members in one study had a longer tenure in the community, participating for a mean of more than 1,000 days (Introne et al., 2016). Periphery members, in contrast, averaged just over 100 days, and extra-periphery members averaged just under 15 days. In other research, participants who were members of more robust communities spent substantially more time participating (Owen, Curran, Bantum, & Hanneman, 2016). The number of connections members had was important in other studies. Members of one health community who continued participating had almost eight times the number of active friends relative to people who discontinued using the community (Stearns et al., 2014). Re-tweeting or forwarding messages related to breast cancer on the microblogging platform Twitter was more common among people who had more followers as well as those who were more central to the network of people discussing breast cancer (Kim, Hou, Han, & Himelboim, 2016).

The importance of one's network or network position extends beyond general participation rates to more specific communication behaviors. In one study, periphery and extra-periphery members were more likely to start a discussion than core members (Introne et al., 2016). Despite their small number, core members made more replies to initial discussion posts compared with periphery and extra-periphery members. Core members were also more likely to share informational support with periphery and extra-periphery members. These findings align with the results from other research in which core or superusers tended to serve as hosts who welcomed new members (Stearns et al., 2014). An analysis of a depression support community in China even showed that network position was associated with microscopic features of messages. Members who were more central to the group tended to write longer messages and were more likely to use second- and third-person personal pronouns (Xu & Zhang, 2016).

A second factor contributing to differences in online health community participation concerns the influence of community members. The nature of a patient's interactions with others in the community can impact the patient's behavior in the community. Members in one smoking cessation community who received a prompt reply to their initial contribution tended to remain a member for a longer period of time (Stearns et al., 2014). In an analysis of an online breast cancer community, members who received a greater number of responses containing emotional support were more likely to remain in the community, whereas those who received more informational support were more likely to leave (Wang, Kraut, & Levine, 2015). The identity of other community members was also important. Online community members were almost twice as likely to contribute to a thread started by a friend rather than one started by a nonfriend, although contribution rates were modest overall (Stearns et al., 2014).

A third factor that can influence participation in online health communities involves homophily, or the tendency for people to associate with similar others. Homophily is particularly important in forming connections. In

SNSs dedicated to weight loss, demographic similarity in terms of age, sex, and health status predicted the likelihood of tie formation (Centola & van de Rijt, 2015; Meng, 2016). Members were more likely to make connections with others who were similar in age, sex, and weight or body mass index. In another study, tie formation based on homophily was observed in start and goal weights (Ma et al., 2010). The influence of homophily extended to the adoption of a health behavior in the form of a diet journal for tracking food consumption (Centola, 2011).

Beyond demographics, homophily based on other factors has been observed. In a study examining conversations about 14 health issues on Twitter, users tended to communicate with others in the same type of health-related role (Xu, Chiu, Chen, & Mukherjee, 2015). Consumers, for example, tended to communicate with other consumers, whereas health care providers communicated with other health providers. In an intervention study, homophily was observed based on the nature of communication technologies used by members (Owen et al., 2016). Members could use one of four different technologies to communicate with one another (e.g., discussion forum, blog, private messages, etc.). Being connected via one technology was associated with having connections via the other communication technologies.

Demographic-related factors are a fourth set of elements that can contribute to differences in online community participation. Research on demographic factors has been largely mixed. Online community members in one study who were older, female, and members for a longer period of time used the community more extensively to connect with others (Cobb et al., 2010). In other research, the number of connections community members had differed by age but not gender or occupation (Urbanoski, van Mierlo, & Cunningham, 2017). Participants who were older had a greater number of connections. Yet other researchers reported no demographic differences in discussion community participation (Selby et al., 2010).

Time is a factor related to demographics that can be important. An analysis of five diabetes mellitus communities showed that time since diagnosis played an important role in community participation (Chomutare, Årsand, Fernandez-Luque, Lauritzen, & Hartvigsen, 2013). Although most community members had been diagnosed within the previous two years, patients who had been diagnosed between two and ten years earlier were most involved in supporting new members. In a mental health online community, the most active and central members were early registrants for the community (Carron-Arthur et al., 2016). Similarly, newer members of a Dutch online health community tended to feel the greatest connection to the community (Tanis, 2008a).

Outcomes of Participation Patterns Participation in health-focused networks online can be consequential. Health behavior (e.g., dieting, exercise, medication adherence) might be considered a complex contagion requiring reinforcement from multiple sources to be adopted (Centola & Macy, 2007). In a social network, reinforcement may take the form of one's connections adopting or advocating the behavior. Several researchers have reported evidence that health behavior acceptance rates increased as a greater number of patients' connections adopted or performed the health behavior.

Studies focusing on weight loss in SNSs (Meng, 2016) and online communities (Ma et al., 2010) have similarly shown that members were significantly more likely to report losing weight when their connections in the network lost weight. Compared to a baseline network, online community members were even more likely to make progress on weight loss when their second- and third-degree friends lost weight (Ma et al., 2010). That is, when their friends' friends or the friends of their friends' friends lost weight, members were more likely to have lost weight relative to the baseline network. In an experimental study, participants were more likely to register for an online community focused on healthy lifestyle behaviors as the number of their connections registered (Centola, 2010). The likelihood of registering increased significantly as a second and third connection in the network registered.

In other research, the amount of exercise performed by users of an activity-tracking SNS was positively associated with the number of connections users had in the community and the amount of exercise performed by their connections (Carpenter & Amaravadi, 2016). Members of the SNS exercised more frequently when they had more connections and their connections engaged in greater levels of exercise. The specific content of messages received from members of one's network also can be consequential. High school students were more likely to report engaging in cigarette smoking or alcohol consumption when a larger number of their offline friends made SNS posts with pictures of "partying" or alcohol consumption (Huang et al., 2014). In a smoking cessation intervention, members who were exposed to group and individual-centric interpersonal messages from other members who had quit smoking were more likely to remain abstinent (Myneni, Fujimoto, Cobb, & Cohen, 2015). Finally, researchers studying an online cancer community found that approximately three-quarters of members exhibited a positive change in the sentiment of their posts as a result of interacting with others in the community (Qiu et al., 2011). As these examples illustrate, the behavior of a patient is influence by the behavior of people with whom the patient is connected.

Network Structure of Online Groups

The structural properties of health-focused groups that appear in online communities, blogs, or other technologies can also be consequential. There is some basic evidence that health communities are unlike online communities formed around different topics such as politics. In one study, message replies in health groups were less equally distributed than in a similar sample of political communities (Himelboim, 2008). That is, health discussion communities were more likely to be marked by a few people making most of the contributions than were political discussion communities. Other researchers have examined the evolution of health-focused online communities. In one study of an online cancer community over an eight-year period, researchers identified three evolutionary sages (Durant, McCray, & Safran, 2010). The first stage, which lasted approximately 20 months, was marked by slow growth. The second stage consisted of a transitional period that lasted approximately one year. In the third stage, rapid growth occurred as the number of members and network activity increased substantially and stabilized.

Online health communities tend to consist of centralized networks with densely connected cores (Introne et al., 2016). A community dedicated to problem alcohol consumption consisted of a dense core and no subgroups (Urbanoski et al., 2017). An online community focused on psychosis was similarly centralized with seven individuals responsible for approximately one-fifth of all links (H.-J. Chang, 2009). This centralization, however, may not extend beyond online communities. Health discussions on the microblogging platform Twitter tended to be decentralized (Xu et al., 2015). No one individual or group dominated the discussions, and the networks lacked a dense core. Researchers have also found distinct networks existing within a single online health community based on discussion topic.

In a community dedicated to skin cancer, the network of members discussing interleukin-2 (IL-2), which tends to be prescribed to people with advanced melanoma, was different from the broader community in several ways (Durant et al., 2010). The IL-2 network was three times as dense as the broader community, and members were more likely to ask questions and receive answers.

There also can be differences in network structure based on the nature of the communication technologies available and used within a community. Participants in one online intervention had access to four different communication technologies, including a discussion forum, blog, e-mail, and a 90-minute weekly chat (Owen et al., 2016). Several trends were observed in the structure of the networks formed across the four technologies. Clustering, which involves the degree to which one's ties are connected with one another, was lowest in e-mail and highest in chat. Path length, reflecting the distance between two people in the network, was notably longer in e-mail than the other three technologies. These results suggest that the networks formed in chat, discussion boards, and blogs were more robust than those found in e-mail. In a smoking cessation intervention, differences in network structure were examined across four technologies, including profile posts, discussion forums, blogs, and private messages similar to e-mail (Zhao et al., 2016). The networks formed using blogs and profile posts were most similar and robust, followed by those formed in the discussion forum. The networks formed using private messaging had the fewest connections, were least dense, and had the greatest path length. Taken together, these two studies suggest that communication technologies allowing asynchronous interactions between dyads tend to be used to construct networks that are not densely connected.

There is also evidence that the structural properties of networks can play a role in health behavior. In one experimental study, participants were randomly assigned to an online community containing a clustered network with a number of redundant ties or a less dense network, including a greater number of weak ties (Centola, 2010). Participants' adoption of a health behavior involving registering for an online healthy lifestyle community varied between the two groups. Registration was greater and occurred more quickly in the densely connected network. Other researchers have reported commensurate findings. Participants in one smoking cessation online intervention who were more central to the network were more likely to have abstained from smoking (Zhao et al., 2016). The results of these studies underscore the role of social influence in promoting health behaviors online. Dense networks and network centrality may serve to reinforce the importance or potential of a given health behavior.

As a whole, the previously reviewed research offers a fairly clear picture of participation in online health groups. Online communities, in particular, are animated by a few active members and a large number of people who participate infrequently. Although a given community may be used by thousands of people over the course of several years, a relatively small proportion tends to contribute most of the content and be most central to the community. Participation in online groups can influence members' health behavior. The adoption or performance of health behaviors is more likely among patients as the number of their connections who have adopted or performed the behavior increases. Finally, online health groups tend to consist of a centralized network with a densely connected core. Network structure, however, can vary based on the nature of the communication technologies used by the group.

Issues Warranting Greater Attention in Research on Making and Reinforcing Connections

Research examining patients' use of communication technologies to make and reinforce social connections has yielded several important insights. Yet questions remain about the implications of communication technologies, and several issues are especially worthy of attention. One issue involves the need for more systematic efforts to study the motivations and outcomes of patients' efforts to connect with others online. Each of the motivations and outcomes identified in this chapter warrants more focused study. Factors driving the various motivations might be considered. Additional research on negative or unintended outcomes similarly would be beneficial. The research reviewed in this chapter suggests that, in some instances, connecting with others online may be counterproductive or even lead to unhealthy behaviors.

A second and related issue that merits greater consideration involves the connections between patients' motivations for using communication technologies and the outcomes of such use. It seems reasonable that patients' motivations could serve to influence the outcomes they experience. In visiting an online community to overcome feelings of isolation, for instance, patients might be particularly likely to identify with community members and perceive their circumstances to not be so extreme. More sophisticated connections between motivations, technology use, and outcomes also might be evaluated. It may be that different types of motivations are connected with different uses of communication technologies such as online communities, which in turn are responsible for specific outcomes.

Beyond further exploring the motivations and outcomes of connecting online, the third and fourth issues meriting greater attention pertain to social networks. Additional research on aggregate participation behavior in health-focused online groups and communities would be valuable. Existing research tends to be consistent with the 1 percent rule and suggests that participation in online communities involves a small proportion of members who contribute most of the content. The implications of this trend are important to evaluate. Beyond considering whether more and less active group members yield different rewards and costs from their participation, it would be valuable to examine group-level outcomes. It seems possible that different types or qualities of resources may be available in communities where participation rates are more evenly distributed. Resources may also covary with the size and density of the network core. It would also be valuable to examine more nuanced differences in participation patterns. Although scholars have begun to consider unique participation styles among online community members (Carron-Arthur, Ali, Cunningham, & Griffiths, 2015), further research is important to identify fundamental differences in participation behavior and the coping implications of such differences.

Finally, researchers would be well served to consider the implications of network structure in online health groups. One avenue would be to further explore the evolution of online health groups such as online communities (Young, 2013). Studies examining how such groups form and are sustained are important. A related practical question involves the optimal structure and dynamics for online communities or SNS. It stands to reason that some structures are likely to yield more benefits for members than others. Identifying those structures and dynamics is an important objective for researchers. A related objective that should be pursued concerns developing design features to enhance the effectiveness of online health groups. It is critical to evaluate those structural or technical elements that could be used to create more robust and helpful online groups for people coping with illness.

Conclusion

Illness can raise the need to connect with other humans. The research reviewed in this chapter suggests the potential of communication technologies for such an endeavor. Several motivations and outcomes of using communication technologies to connect with others were identified. Most notably, communication technologies use is motivated by a desire to overcome feelings of isolation, reach similar others, and bolster patients' existing relationships with friends and family. The most salient outcomes include becoming involved in a community, relief from distress, and, in some cases, increased distress. Several network-related dimensions of making connections also have been considered. In online communities, a small proportion of members tend to be most central to the community and contribute a disproportionally large amount of the content. The vast majority of people who participate do so infrequently and tend to contribute little. More broadly, the networks formed in health groups online such as SNSs and online communities tend to be centralized and contain a dense core. In interpreting these conclusions, it is important to keep in mind that they are drawn from a nascent body of scholarship. Researchers have just begun to examine patients' use of communication technologies for social connection. Additional work is essential to more fully understand the implications of communication technologies for connecting with others and coping with illness digitally.

3 Soliciting and Providing Social Support

Illness can place an incredible strain on a patient's resources (Lyons, Sullivan, Ritvo, & Coyne, 1995). It may result in physical discomfort or pain over prolonged periods of time. Illness may limit one's mobility and make it difficult to complete everyday tasks such as folding laundry or grocery shopping. Even with insurance, illness can create considerable financial difficulties stemming from missed work or the inability to maintain employment. Beyond the physical and financial challenges, illness can tax a patient's sense of well-being and personal relationships. The notion that one is "sick" or "unwell" can erode a patient's sense of self, security, and optimism about the future. Perhaps more than any other time in life, the myriad of challenges posed by illness create a significant need for social support (Cohen, Underwood, & Gottlieb, 2000).

The thesis of this chapter is that communication technologies have important implications for coping with illness by providing opportunities for acquiring and sharing social support. The chapter begins with an overview of the ways in which social support has been proposed to function and studied by scholars. Patients' use of communication technologies for seeking support is then considered, followed by the outcomes of support acquired online. The role of communication technologies in providing social support is evaluated next, along with the content and outcomes of support expression online. The chapter concludes with a discussion of issues that warrant greater attention in scholarship on communication technologies and social support.

Illness and Social Support

Fundamentals of Social Support

Widely accepted to play an integral role in health and coping with illness (Cohen & Wills, 1985; Wills & Ainette, 2012), social support generally involves the implications of social relationships for well-being (Cohen et al., 2000). It has been consistently linked with physical functioning as well as psychological well-being among people coping with illness (Uchino, 2009). Despite agreement about its benefits, social support has been thought about and studied in several different ways. Much of the research in this chapter is grounded in the assumption that social support functions by buffering the effects of health-related stressors. In the stress-buffering model (Cohen & Wills, 1985), social support is proposed to come between a stressor—a specific event such as a health setback or a more chronic concern—and a stress response. Social support can serve to directly reduce patients' distress by helping them directly deal with their issues or by influencing the way they appraise stressors. Both effects serve to lessen the negative impact of stress on health. The buffering model has been shown to offer one reasonable explanation for the benefits of social support (Wills & Ainette, 2012).

Another important distinction involves how social support has been studied (Gottlieb & Bergen, 2010). Social support has been examined in terms of the perception that, if necessary, one has people available who could be called on for assistance (i.e., perceived support availability). A great deal of evidence links perceived support with coping efforts and health outcomes (Wethington & Kessler, 1986; Wills & Shinar, 2000). A related approach for examining social support involves considering the number of supportive messages or acts one receives during a given time period (i.e., received support). The benefits of received support have been much more difficult to demonstrate in empirical research (Bolger, Zuckerman, & Kessler, 2000). Although receiving physical assistance or having someone listen to one's problems would intuitively seem to be helpful, a number of studies have shown no or even negative effects stemming from received support (Wills & Shinar, 2000).

A third, distinct approach for studying social support involves focusing on the content of messages produced in attempts to provide support. This work is represented by scholars who have sought to catalog messages containing different types of support (Cutrona & Suhr, 1992; House, 1980). Beyond developing typologies, researchers have focused on better understanding the characteristics of helpful support messages. Efforts have been made to isolate the rhetorical moves and linguistic features of comforting messages (Burleson, 1994), advice (MacGeorge, Feng, Butler, & Budarz, 2004), and messages that attempt to bolster receivers' self-esteem (Holmstrom & Burleson, 2011).

Affordances of Communication Technologies for Social Support

Four affordances of communication technologies are particularly relevant to social support, including control, anonymity, visibility, and availability. These affordances represent dimensions of communication technologies that can be salient in the processes of acquiring and sharing social support. Each factor is identified in table 3.1 and will be considered in the following paragraphs.

The affordance of control involves the potential to manage aspects of human interaction, such as the ability to edit a message prior to when it is shared. Relative to face-to-face conversations, asynchronous communication technologies that allow for a delay between when a message is sent and received (e.g., online support communities, blogs) typically offer greater interactional control. This affordance may be used by support seekers to feel more comfortable in seeking assistance (Rains & Keating, 2011; Walther & Boyd, 2002). Particularly in the context of illness, needing and requesting assistance can be seen as a sign of weakness—that one is unable or unwilling to meet one's challenges. The asynchronous nature of message exchange can be used to make such requests easier by allowing them to be carefully crafted. Control can make it possible for support seekers to better protect their dignity when requesting help.

Table 3.1

Key Affordances of Communication Technologies for Social Support

Affordance	Definition
Control	Potential to manage aspects of interaction related to message construction and sharing.
Anonymity	Potential to conceal one's identity.
Visibility	Potential to be seen by others or observe others' behavior.
Availability	Potential to access resources when they are most needed.

Anonymity is a second affordance of communication technologies important for seeking support (Tanis, 2008b; Walther & Boyd, 2002; Wright & Bell, 2003). Anonymity involves concealing one's identity from others. A pseudonym may be used in an online support community, for example, or one's legal name may otherwise be withheld. This affordance can function to mitigate a support seeker's fear of retribution or potential to be held accountable for his or her requests. In the context of illness, where stigma is a pervasive concern (Scambler, 2009), being able to conceal one's identity can allow people to feel less wary of making support requests than when their identity is known. One can discuss and ask for help about embarrassing or controversial issues with less concern about retribution.

Visibility is a third affordance that has implications for support seeking. Visibility involves the degree to which one's behavior is observable or others' behavior can be observed. Blogs and social network sites (SNSs) may allow support seekers to signal a need for assistance to potentially vast audiences of would-be support providers (Rains & Wright, 2016). These technologies also make it possible for support seekers to observe others facing similar challenges. Being able to witness how others deal with a particular issue or the consequences of other patients' behavior can be a valuable coping resource.

A final affordance of communication technologies relevant to social support is availability or the potential to connect with support providers when they are most needed (Walther & Boyd, 2002; Wright & Bell, 2003). Unlike a formal health care provider, such as a medical doctor, several communication technologies offer immediate access to potential support resources. Online support communities, for example, do not require an appointment and are available virtually any time of the day and every day of the year. Support seekers can seek assistance as soon as the need arises.

Seeking Social Support Online

With a basic understanding of what social support is and the relevant technological affordances, it is important to next consider the ways in which communication technologies are used to acquire support. Although it may be surprising today, researchers studying the Internet and computer-mediated communication (CMC) during the 1980s and early 1990s initially questioned the potential for people to form meaningful social relationships when using computers to communicate. The cues-filtered-out perspective (Culnan & Markus, 1987) summarized several theories and predicted that the reduction in social cues stemming from the inability to see one's interaction partner or hear his or her voice would lead to less personal exchanges than in face-to-face interactions. As such, Internet users would be both unmotivated and unable to provide effective support. For example, Kiesler, Siegel, and McGuire (1984) conducted a series of experiments and found evidence that, relative to groups meeting face to face, computer-mediated groups were much more likely to engage in antisocial behavior in the form of profanity, insults, and name calling. Despite such findings, they also saw promise in CMC. In discussing directions for future research, they proposed that, "It might be possible to turn computer networks into social support networks" (Kiesle et al., 1984, p. 1131).

Since Kiesler and colleagues' (1984) seminal work, a substantial number of U.S. adults have used the Internet for seeking support to cope with illness. The almost 5 million U.S. adults estimated to have used an online support community dedicated to a health condition or personal problem by 2000 (Fox & Rainie, 2000) grew to approximately 31 million Internet users who had tried to locate others facing similar health concerns as of 2012 (Fox & Duggan, 2013). Yet relatively little is known about the demographic characteristics of online support seekers. Researchers examining online peer support for mental health have found that support seekers were more likely to be female, be White, and have a college education (DeAndrea & Anthony, 2013). Females, Whites, and those with higher levels of distress were also more likely to seek support online compared with those attending a face-to-face support group (DeAndrea, 2015). Other researchers examining the demographic characteristics of online cancer community members have found that members were middle-age and more likely to be women, and almost half were college graduates (Im et al., 2007). Notably, cancer stages one through four were all fairly well represented, with most respondents facing stage two.

Patients may acquire social support in a number of settings online. Studies with nationally representative samples (Hampton, Goulet, Rainie, & Purcell, 2011) and undergraduate samples (Liu & LaRose, 2008) showed that Internet use is generally associated with perceived support availability. These findings extend to specific communication technologies. SNS users reported greater levels of support availability than nonusers (Hampton et al., 2011), and time spent playing massively multiplayer online games (MMOGs) was positively associated with support available from other game players (Kaczmarek & Krazkowski, 2014; Longman, O'Connor, & Obst, 2009). In health-related settings, blogging frequency involving the number of posts made or time spent blogging was positively associated with perceptions of support availability in general (McDaniel, Coyne, & Holmes, 2012) as well as specifically from bloggers' blog readers (Rains & Keating, 2011). These findings can be contrasted with studies showing no association between perceptions of support availability and support-related Internet use (Eastin & LaRose, 2005) or SNS use (McDaniel et al., 2012). In one study examining the implications of individual technologies within online health communities, use of the discussion board was positively associated with patients' perceptions of emotional and informational support available from community members (Chung, 2014). Photo/video sharing and blog use, however, were not associated with support availability perceptions.

Less is known about the implications of communication technology use for received support. Time spent using online communities dedicated to HIV/AIDS (Mo & Coulson, 2013) and weight loss (Hwang et al., 2011) has been shown to be positively associated with informational and emotional support received from the community. Yet women coping with infertility reported receiving significantly less support than they desired from online sources (High & Steuber, 2014). This trend in unsatisfactory support, however, extended to medical professionals and other support sources such as spouses.

Other researchers showed that the type of support received depended on contextual factors such as patients' motivations for using communication technologies or illness stage. Among members of an online infertility community, those who joined to exchange information reported receiving greater levels of emotional and informational support (Welbourne, Blanchard, & Wadsworth, 2013). Yet joining to exchange emotional support was not associated with support received. In a smoking cessation online community, informational support tended to flow to people early in their quit attempt from people in later quit stages (Zhang & Yang, 2015). Nurturant forms of support, such as emotional support, followed the same trend but were also exchanged by people within a given quit stage. The nature of patients' connections in a network is another important factor.

Researchers examining a weight loss SNS found that network closure, which involves having connections to people who are connected to one another (e.g., having two friends who are also friends with one another), was associated with receiving a greater volume of emotional and esteems support messages (Meng, Chung, & Cox, 2016). Network brokerage, which involves having connections to people who are not connected to one another, was associated with receiving a greater volume of informational, network, and emotional support messages.

Taken as a whole, some conclusions can be drawn about support seeking online. The Internet has become a widely used resource for seeking support. Use of various technologies from blogs to SNSs is connected with perceptions of support availability. Given the cross-sectional nature of most research on this topic, however, it is difficult to determine the causal nature of this association. It is unclear whether patients with greater support available are drawn to seek support online or whether using these technologies is responsible for increasing support available to patients—or both. The implications of communication technologies for received support are not well understood. It appears that contextual factors may play a role in determining the types of support that patients receive online.

The Outcomes of Support Available and Received Online

Having discussed the potential of communication technologies to serve as support resources, it is important to consider the outcomes of online support. Social support acquired or available online can have important implications for patients' coping efforts. The outcomes of perceived and received support will be examined in the following section. The implications of patients' offline support resources and the potential of support interventions for promoting patients' health and well-being will then be evaluated.

Support Received and Available Online

A fair amount of agreement exists among researchers about why support received and available online might be beneficial to patients. Much of the work in this area is grounded—whether explicitly or implicitly—in ideas from the buffering model (Cohen & Wills, 1985). Received and perceived support are thought to directly mitigate a source of distress and/or reduce a patient's appraisal of stressor severity or enhance perceptions of their cop-ing efforts (Lakey & Cohen, 2000). Through helping patients to directly address a problem or by changing the way they think about the problem, perceived and received support can promote patient well-being.

Support available online has been shown to be a valuable resource. Indeed, the benefits of available support have been documented in online communities (Mo & Coulson, 2010, 2013; Oh & Lee, 2012), SNSs (Liu & Yu, 2013; Oh, Ozkaya, & LaRose, 2014; Wright et al., 2013), blogs (Ko & Kuo, 2009; Rains & Keating, 2011), microblogs (Liang, Ho, Li, & Turban, 2011), and MMOGs (Kaczmarek & Krazkowski, 2014; Longman et al., 2009). Although most of the preceding studies do not focus specifically on patients, a few have demonstrated the potential benefits of support avail-ability among this group. Perceptions of support available from members of a diabetes support community (Oh & Lee, 2012) and health bloggers' readers (Rains & Keating, 2011) were positively associated with perceptions of health-related empowerment. The availability of specific types of sup-port has also been shown to be valuable. Emotional support available from members of undergraduate students' SNS networks was associated with greater levels of health self-efficacy (Oh, Lauckner, Boehmer, Fewins-Bliss, & Li, 2013). Similarly, the availability of emotional support was associated with greater levels of physical, psychological, and existential quality of life in an online hepatitis community (Yao, Zheng, & Fan, 2015). Informational support availability, however, was only associated with greater levels of physical quality of life.

The potential effects of support received online are less clear. The results of studies examining overall levels of support received from SNS networks are inconsistent (H. Kim, 2014; Oh et al., 2014). Yet evaluations of spe-cific support types have been more promising. Emotional support, which involves comforting and understanding, has been shown to be beneficial in a few studies (Kim et al., 2012; Turner et al., 2013; Vlahovic, Wang, Kraut, & Levine, 2014). In one particularly impressive study, Turner and colleagues (2013) examined 618 e-mail messages sent over the course of six months from health care providers to 41 patients diagnosed with type 1 or type 2 diabetes for the presence of emotional support messages. They also evalu-ated patients' HbA1c levels, which is an indicator of glycemic control, at the beginning and end of the six-month period. The proportion of emo-tional support messages sent from health care providers to patients was associated with changes in patients' HbA1c levels. Patients who received more emotional support from their health care provider were more likely to experience improved physiological functioning in the form of glycemic control.

In other research, women in breast cancer support communities who received more emotional support messages reported lower levels of breast cancer concerns (Kim et al., 2012). Yet in two additional studies, the benefits of receiving emotional support for breast cancer concerns were limited to women with moderate and high levels of emotional communication competence (Yoo et al., 2014) or who provided high levels of emotional support to other community members (Han et al., 2012). The outcomes of receiving support also appear to depend on the types of support sought. When support seekers in one breast cancer online community solicited informational support, receiving emotional support was associated with less satisfaction and receiving informational support was associated with greater satisfaction (Vlahovic et al., 2014). No such trend was observed when emotional support was sought.

There is also reason to believe that individual-difference factors may play a role in who most benefits from online support. Wright's (Wright & Miller, 2010; Wright, Rains, & Banas, 2010) notion of preference for support from weak ties is rooted in broader ideas about the function of weak ties in social networks (Granovetter, 1973). Among patients, weak ties consist of peers with whom patients do not share a close relationship but from whom they can acquire resources. Wright contends that some patients may have an enduring preference for support from weak ties because they are less risky disclosure targets, present less potential for role conflict, and can provide novel information (Wright & Miller, 2010). In studies of online health community members, preference for weak-tie support was negatively related to anxiety (Wright & Miller, 2010) and stress (Wright et al., 2010). Wright and Rains (2013) argued that the support acquired from an online community would be more beneficial to patients who preferred support from weak ties. They surveyed members of health-related online support communities and found that the associations between stigma and two negative outcomes were weaker among patients who had a greater preference for weak ties relative to patients who had less of a preference for weak-tie support. In other words, the deleterious effects of stigma were not as strong among online community members who had a greater preference for weak ties.

Offline Support

Several scholars have argued that online sources of social support may be particularly valuable when one's traditional support sources, such as family and friends, are unable or unwilling to provide assistance (Tanis, 2008a; Wright & Bell, 2003). Turner, Grube, and Meyers (2001) adapted the concept of support matching—in which the most beneficial outcomes are proposed to occur when the type of support is matched to the nature of the stressor faced by a support seeker (Cutrona, 1990; Cutrona & Russell, 1990)—to explain when and why online support could be particularly valuable. They argued that online support sources may be able to meet the needs of patients when their offline support sources such as friends or family are unable or unwilling to provide effective support. Because online support sources are often coping with the same health condition as those patients seeking support, they are uniquely situated to meet patients' needs for information and understanding. Kraut and colleagues' (2002) social compensation hypothesis is based on a similar premise. Internet use is proposed to have differential consequences based on one's access to offline support and social resources. Social compensation occurs as individuals "with fewer social resources [...] use the new communication opportunities on-line to form connections with people and obtain supportive communication and useful information otherwise missing locally" (Kraut et al., 2002, p. 58).

Taken together, the matching model (Turner et al., 2001) and social compensation hypothesis (Kraut et al., 2002) both suggest that seeking support online should allow individuals to better meet their unique support needs and overcome support deficits in offline relationships. Some initial evidence for this idea has been found (Cummings, Sproull, & Kiesler, 2002). Turner and colleagues (2001), for example, surveyed a sample of online support community members and found that, among members who lacked depth in a significant offline relationship, time spent in the community and e-mail contact with members was positively associated with the depth of their relationship with the community. That is, among people who lacked support offline, those who participated in the community more frequently reported a greater connection to the community. Another group of scholars surveyed a sample of health bloggers and found that the support bloggers perceived available from their readers was most consequential to those bloggers who lacked support from their friends and family (Rains &

Keating, 2011). When friend and family support was low, bloggers who had greater levels of support available online reported less loneliness and greater personal growth resulting from illness.

Evidence also indicates that people with the greatest offline resources may be most drawn to and benefit from online support. Kraut and colleagues (2002) conducted a longitudinal study and found that Internet use was associated with increased family interaction among individuals who reported greater levels of support availability. The benefits of Internet use for connecting with family were most substantial among individuals who already perceived higher levels of support available. In other research, people who perceived more support available from their friends and family evaluated online health communities more positively (Ruppel & McKinley, 2015), and those with more cohesive family situations made greater use of an online breast cancer community (Yoo et al., 2014). Finally, in a study of support received using a popular SNS, the responses that participants identified as most supportive were more likely to come from one of their close relationships than from an acquaintance (Blight, Jagiello, & Ruppel, 2015).

Support Interventions

Social support has also played an important role in Internet-based interventions developed for people coping with various health conditions. The interventions are delivered by medical professionals and restricted to patients coping with a specific condition who have been recruited to participate. They tend to be conducted on a website developed specifically for the intervention. Although variation exists among individual Internet-based interventions, most tend to include an educational component and a group communication component. Most relevant to this chapter, such interventions include an online discussion community where patients can interact with other patients participating in the intervention. The utility of these interventions has been demonstrated in several studies. In one meta-analysis, which is a method of summarizing the results from existing quantitative studies, 28 interventions involving more than 4,000 participants were examined (Rains & Young, 2009). Each intervention focused on one health condition, such as depression (Gerrits, van der Zanden, Visscher, & Conijn, 2007), breast cancer (Gustafson et al., 2005), cardiovascular disease (LaCoursiere, 2001), or diabetes (McKay, Glasgow, Feil, Boles, & Barrera,

2002). From the beginning of the interventions to completion, the average participant experienced increased levels of social support, self-efficacy, and quality of life as well as decreased depression.

Several moderating factors related to the group communication component served to strengthen or weaken the effects of the interventions (Rains & Young, 2009). Relative to patients who had access to only asynchronous communication technologies such as a discussion board, patients in interventions that also included synchronous technologies, such as instant messaging, experienced greater increases in social support. The findings also offered tentative evidence that patients in interventions lasting a greater number of weeks experienced larger gains in social support. Finally, patients in larger discussion groups experienced increased quality of life but also decreased social support. Taken as a whole, these results offer evidence that the group communication component of computer-mediated support interventions was consequential for patients—particularly for social support. More communication technologies and time for relationships to develop were both linked with greater increases in social support from the baseline to intervention completion. Yet discussion groups that were too large appeared to create difficulties for making connections and acquiring support.

The Implications of CMC for Support Processes

Although support available and received online can be beneficial for patients, the role of computer mediation has received comparatively little attention. Yet e-mail, instant messaging, and contemporary forms of social media such as SNSs and blogs all involve CMC. Understanding the implications of those basic properties that define CMC for supportive interaction is critical to fully realize the potential of communication technologies for social support. Theoretical explanations for the effects of CMC are discussed next, followed by empirical research examining this issue.

Theoretical Explanations

One pressing question for researchers studying social support online involves the consequences of CMC for supportive interactions. As previously discussed, CMC is different from face-to-face interaction in a few important ways. One difference involves the reduction in social cues stemming from text-based forms of interaction. It is not possible to make eye contact, see facial expressions, or hear others' voices during CMC. Walther and Parks (2002) refer to this reduction in social cues as one of two "structural aspects of social support" that are "fundamentally changed" by CMC (p. 545). A second difference involves the potential for asynchronous interaction. In CMC a delay can occur between when messages are sent and received.

Two primary theories have been invoked in considering the implications of CMC for social support processes. Walther's (1996) hyperpersonal communication model has been used to make predictions about the way in which CMC impacts a support seeker and provider's perceptions of one another during supportive interaction. The hyperpersonal model has four components that serve to explain how CMC can be more personal than face-to-face interaction. Senders engage in strategic self-presentation and present themselves in the most positive light possible, while receivers use this information in the absence of visual and vocal cues to develop idealized perceptions of senders. The asynchronous nature of CMC and feedback processes also contributes to the hyperpersonal effect. Wright and Bell (2003) proposed that hyperpersonal communication could happen among patients in online support contexts. Online support community members, for example, may perceive one another to be especially close and idealize the support they receive in this environment.

A second theoretical approach for understanding the implications of CMC for social support involves the theory of conversationally induced reappraisals (Burleson & Goldsmith, 1998). The process of reappraising an upsetting experience—in which we come to see the stressor as less problematic or more manageable—is central to comforting communication. A number of rhetorical moves argued to facilitate reappraisal are identified in the theory. Caplan and Turner (2007) argued that CMC may facilitate comforting communication and the reappraisal process. Relative to face-to-face interaction, they argued that CMC creates a safer conversational environment where support seekers feel comfortable discussing distressing issues, fosters empathy among support providers and allows them to focus the discussion on the support seeker's feelings, and encourages support seekers to express personal narratives about their upsetting experiences. These three factors are proposed to help nurture the reappraisal process and, ultimately, lead to more helpful supportive interactions.

Empirical Research

Research testing the unique implications of CMC for social support processes has tended to focus on examining the effects of those social cues that persist online. Identity information about support seekers and providers revealed in screen names and avatars can have important consequences for supportive interaction. In one study, participants judged a hypothetical supportive interaction from an online support community in which the nature of the support message and the sex of the support provider were manipulated (Spottswood, Walther, Holmstrom, & Ellison, 2013). Relative to when the support provider had a female or ambiguous sex name, male participants liked and perceived more effective messages involving high levels of person-centeredness when the support provider had a male name. Person-centeredness involves recognizing and legitimizing the feelings of others (MacGeorge, Feng, & Burleson, 2011). Female participants' perceptions were not impacted by the sex of the support provider. In other experimental research, participants were asked to serve as support providers and write a response to a request for support ostensibly appearing in an online community (Feng, Li, & Li, 2016). Participants wrote more person-centered and polite support messages when a picture and first name (e.g., Will) was used by support seekers than when there was no picture and a non-name screen name (e.g., WR10) was used.

In addition to specific cues related to identity, more subtle features of interaction can impact support processes online. The number of features used in conveying emotional distress was examined in one study (High, Oeldorf-Hirsh, & Bellur, 2014). Contrary to what might be expected, participants were less willing to provide emotional and network support when multiple features of an SNS were used to convey distress (i.e., status message, relationship feature, profile picture) than when one feature was used. Time is another subtle feature of interaction that can be important. Relative to when the time delay between an e-mail support request and response was one month, neutral observers rated support providers as more immediate and receptive when the delay was one hour (Ledbetter, 2008). These results were partially replicated in a second study where females rated the e-mail support message more positively when the delay was shorter.

Interpersonal coordination has also been shown to be consequential. Language style matching is a form of interpersonal coordination that involves the degree to which two speakers match one another's use of function words such as prepositions, adverbs, and pronouns (Ireland

& Pennebaker, 2010). Because they require shared knowledge to use and understand, function words reflect and foster rapport. In one study, language style matching between health bloggers and their readers (in the comments they left on the blog) over the course of a three-month period was examined as a predictor of bloggers' perceptions of support available from readers (Rains, 2016). When language style matching between health bloggers and their readers increased, bloggers reported perceiving greater levels of emotional support available from readers. There was also tentative evidence of a connection between language style matching and bloggers' perceptions of informational support available from readers. Taken as whole, the results of research examining identity and interactional features indicate that, despite the reduction in social cues, subtle aspects of CMC can contribute to perceptions of support providers and interactions.

Beyond subtle features of interaction, there appear to be differences in the nature and outcomes of supportive communication occurring face to face and via CMC. A few researchers have documented the benefits of CMC. In a cross-sectional study of counseling meetings, participants who communicated with their counselor via CMC reported more effective interactions relative to participants who interacted with their counselor face to face (Cook & Doyle, 2002). In another study, undergraduate students completed a formal counseling session about anxiety run by a graduate student in counseling psychology (Cohen & Kerr, 1999). Although no differences occurred between the face-to-face and instant messaging groups regarding participants' perceptions of the counselor or the interaction, participants reported lower levels of arousal in the CMC condition.

Use of CMC for supportive interactions has also been linked to less beneficial outcomes relative to face-to-face communication. In a cross-sectional study, current and former military members were asked to evaluate the level of disruption caused by a negative life event and the nature of the communication technology they used to acquire event-related support (Lewandowski, Rosenberg, Parks, & Siegel, 2011). Participants who primarily received face-to-face support experienced more improvement than those who received support via CMC. In an experimental study, High and Solomon (2014) randomly assigned participants to provide high, medium, or low levels of person-centered support to a friend either face to face or via instant messaging. Support providers in the instant messaging condition reported lower levels of self-presentational confidence. Moreover, two weeks after the supportive interaction, females who received low person-centered support in the instant messaging condition reported less improvement in their problem than women who received low person-centered face-to-face support. In another experiment, participants interacted with a confederate who provided support face to face or via instant messaging (Rains, Brunner, Akers, Pavlich, & Goktas, 2017). Participants were asked a series of questions designed to make the stress of finding a job after graduation salient and then received social support. Relative to the face-to-face condition, the discussion left participants in the instant messaging condition more worried and uncomfortable with their uncertainty about finding a job.

The previously reviewed research invites substantially different conclusions about the consequences of CMC for supportive interactions. CMC has been shown to foster more and less beneficial support outcomes relative to face-to-face communication. In an effort to reconcile these discrepant findings, one group of researchers sought to isolate the implications of CMC specifically for support message processing (Rains, Brunner, Akers, Pavlich, & Tsetsi, 2016). Drawing from the dual-process theory of supportive message outcomes (Bodie & Burleson, 2008), they argued that the reduced social cues associated with CMC have the potential to impact a support seeker's ability and motivation to receive support, and thereby enhance the effects of support messages relative to face-to-face interaction. The reduction in social cues can make CMC less taxing on a support seeker's attentional resources. Support seekers do not have to worry about managing nonverbal behavior such as facial expressions and eye contact as one might during face-to-face interaction. As such, support seekers should have greater ability to receive support in CMC and be more likely to focus on their stressor, which could serve to increase their motivation to receive support. The researchers argued that increased motivation and ability would encourage support seekers to more closely attend to a support message in CMC and bolster its effects compared with face-to-face interaction.

To test this idea, the researchers conducted an experiment in which participants were asked to discuss a relevant stressor with a confederate (Rains et al., 2016). The interaction took place face to face, via instant messaging, or via instant messaging while completing a simple counting task designed to (slightly) restrict participants' attentional resources. The researchers reasoned that, if the reduced demands for attentional resources in CMC were key, then participants who performed the attention-taxing task while using instant messaging should experience outcomes commensurate with the face-to-face group. Notably, participants in all conditions received the exact same support message from the confederate—the only difference between the conditions was the nature of the communication medium. The results were fairly consistent with expectations. Relative to the face-to-face or CMC condition with the attention-taxing task, participants in the CMC condition were most motivated to receive support, processed the support message most extensively, and experienced the most adaptive changes in uncertainty about the stressor as a result of the interaction.

The findings from this study offer evidence that CMC alone does not make supportive interactions any better or worse than face-to-face communication (Rains et al., 2016). Rather, the reduced social cues in CMC impact support seekers' motivation to receive support, elaboration on support messages received, and ultimately bolster the effects of those messages. Although a relatively high-quality support message was used in their study and subsequently produced beneficial effects, it is equally likely that a low-quality support message would foster more negative outcomes in CMC relative to face-to-face interaction—as has been found in previous research (High & Solomon, 2014).

A few conclusions may be drawn from theory and research involving the effects of CMC on support processes and outcomes. Despite the potential of theories such as the hyperpersonal model and theory of conversationally induced reappraisals, few studies have been undertaken to test these ideas in the context of computer-mediated support. The empirical research conducted indicates that subtle social cues online can impact perceptions of support providers and messages. The consequences of CMC for social support relative to face-to-face communication are not well understood. CMC has been shown to have both positive and negative implications for supportive interactions. Initial evidence suggests that CMC may function to encourage greater attention to support messages.

The Content and Outcomes of Support Expression Online

A final area of research on communication technologies and social support involves support provision. The content of support messages shared in various health contexts online will be addressed, followed by the consequences of support provision for the provider. The chapter concludes with a discussion of some issues that warrant greater attention in research on social support and communication technologies.

The Content of Support Messages Shared Online

A great deal has been learned about the types of support messages patients send and receive online. Much of the research in this area involves categorizing the messages shared in a context such as online support communities dedicated to a specific health issue such as infertility (Malik & Coulson, 2008), depression (Keating, 2013), or cancer (Ginossar, 2008). Although considerably less prevalent, a few researchers have also examined other online settings such as blogs (Tong, Heinemann-LaFave, Jeon, Kolodziej-Smith, & Warshay, 2013) and microblogs (Turner-McGrievy & Tate, 2013). The messages appearing in these contexts are typically assigned to one of several categories corresponding to different types of social support. Cutrona and Suhr's (1992) social support behavior code (SSBC) is a frequently used coding scheme. It contains five categories of support: informational, emotional, esteem, network, and tangible. The full coding scheme is presented in table 3.2. In brief, informational support involves advice or facts, whereas emotional support consists of comforting and attempts to demonstrate caring. Esteem support includes efforts to bolster one's self-concept, and network support involves attempts to increase one's social network or communicate belonging. Finally, tangible support includes offers of physical assistance, such as help with housework.

A meta-analysis of 41 original studies showed several trends in the prevalence of different support message types shared among patients in contexts such as online support communities (Rains, Peterson, & Wright, 2015). Informational and emotional support were much more common than the other types of support messages. They were also the only two types of messages appearing more frequently than would be expected by chance. Esteem and network support messages were less prevalent than informational and emotional support messages and less common than would be expected by chance. Tangible support messages were the least common of all support message types.

The results of this meta-analysis offer several insights about how communication technologies such as online communities are being used by patients as a coping resource. Informational and emotional support, which were far and away the most common types of support, are noteworthy in

Table 3.2
Cutrona and Suhr's (1992) SSBC Framework for Identifying Support Messages

SSBC Support Type	Purpose of Message
Informational support	
Advice	Offers ideas and suggests actions
Referral	Refers the recipient to some other source of help
Situation appraisal	Reassesses or redefines the situation
Teaching	Provides detailed information, facts, or news about the situation or about skills needed to deal with the situation
Tangible assistance	
Loan	Offers to lend the recipient something
Direct task	Offers to perform a task directly related to the stress
Indirect task	Offers to take over one or more of the recipient's other responsibilities while the recipient is under stress
Active participation	Offers to join the recipient in action that reduces the stress
Willingness	Expresses willingness to help
Esteem support	
Compliment	Says positive things about the recipient or emphasizes the recipient's abilities
Validation	Expresses agreement with the recipient's perspective on the situation
Relief of blame	Tries to alleviate the recipient's feelings of guilt about the situation
Network support	
Access	Offers to provide the recipient with access to new companions
Presence	Offers to spend time with the person
Companions	Reminds the recipient of availability of companions such as others who are similar in interests or experiences
Emotional support	
Relationship	Stresses the importance of closeness and love in relationship with the recipient
Physical affection	Offers physical contact, including hugs, kisses, hand-holding, shoulder patting
Confidentiality	Promises to keep the recipient's problem in confidence

Table 3.2 (continued)

SSBC Support Type	Purpose of Message
Sympathy	Expresses sorrow or regret for the recipient's situation or distress
Listening	Makes attentive comments as the recipient speaks
Empathy	Expresses understanding of the situation or discloses a personal situation that communicates understanding
Encouragement	Provides the recipient with hope and confidence
Prayer	Prays with the recipient

that they directly align with problem- and emotion-focused coping (Lazarus & Folkman, 1984). Informational support facilitates problem-focused coping by providing advice, feedback, and situation appraisals that make it possible to take action and address a stressor. Emotional support aids emotion-focused coping by attempting to help people deal with the aversive feelings associated with a stressor. Messages that communicate caring and understanding can help alleviate distress, which is central to emotion-focused coping efforts. Although significantly less common, communication technologies such as online communities also provide a resource for expanding one's social network and bolstering one's self-worth. Unsurprisingly, tangible support was relatively uncommon. This finding underscores the limits of acquiring support in contexts such as online communities. Despite being a valuable resource for information or comfort, these contexts have limited potential to produce physical assistance, such as help with household chores.

The Outcomes of Providing Social Support

Researchers have just begun to consider the potential consequences of providing social support online for the support provider. Most of the work in this area has been conducted in the context of support interventions for women with breast cancer and is limited to the provision of emotional support (Han et al., 2012; Kim et al., 2011, 2012; Yoo et al., 2014). Computerized content analysis was used in these works to capture explicit emotional support message that take forms such as, "Sorry to hear about … ," "My heart goes out to you … ," and "You have my sympathy. …" A positive association was found in one study between the provision and receipt of emotional support (Kim et al., 2012). Patients who received more emotional support messages also provided a greater number of support messages to others. The basic connection between providing and receiving support has also been observed in informal online health communities (Welbourne et al., 2013). One explanation for this phenomenon is the norm of reciprocity, which dictates that those who receive support from others may feel compelled to provide support.

The provision of emotional support by patients has been linked with positive outcomes, including positive reframing (Kim et al., 2011, 2012) and reduced self-blame (Kim et al., 2011). Patients who were more likely to provide support had a greater tendency to positively reframe their situation and engage in less self-blame. One explanation for the benefits of providing support to other patients involves the idea that providing support is an act of "self-persuasion" that is empowering because it involves self-reflection (Kim et al., 2012). Another possibility is that support provision allows patients to learn new coping skills or become aware of a different perspective (Kim et al., 2012).

Research on support provision has not been uniformly positive. In one study, support provision was associated with higher levels of perceived stress (Welbourne et al., 2013). Other researchers have found that the effects of support provision depend on certain factors. Providing emotional support was associated with greater quality of life among patients who had higher levels of emotional competence (Yoo et al., 2014) and reduced breast cancer concerns among patients who received high levels of emotional support (Han et al., 2012). Clearly, additional research would be valuable to better understand the implications of providing support online for support providers.

Issues Warranting Greater Attention in Social Support Research

Although a great deal of progress has occurred in research examining the implications of communication technologies for social support among patients, several issues should be privileged in future scholarship. First, this body of research would benefit from a greater focus on applying, developing, and refining theory related to social support, communication technologies, and coping with illness. Walther's (1996) hyperpersonal communication model, for example, is fairly frequently invoked in research on this topic but is rarely explicitly tested. It would be valuable to directly examine the implications of this and related theories in the context of supportive interactions. It is possible that, relative to face-to-face interaction, support providers could have exaggerated impressions of support seekers, which in turn may impact the relative quality of the supportive messages they produce. Beyond further studying existing theories and models, it would be valuable to consider those affordances frequently identified as playing an important role in support processes. Relatively little research has been conducted to directly consider the consequences of anonymity, availability, control, and other affordances for using communication technologies to seek support and the specific nature of support-seeking efforts.

A second issue meriting greater attention involves the outcomes of supportive interaction in computer-mediated contexts. Much of the research examining support outcomes related to well-being has tended to focus on perceived support availability. Although support availability is important to consider, additional research examining received support would be valuable. It is critical to better understand the specific types of support patients are acquiring online and the role that it plays in coping efforts. Initial evidence indicates that emotional support received online can be beneficial. The effects of other support types deserve to be studied. Research examining the potential benefits of support provision for support providers would also be valuable. Moreover, the role of CMC in bringing about such effects needs greater attention.

A third and related series of issues that deserve greater attention involve support provision online. Although research has been conducted to better understand the prevalence of different types of support messages shared in health contexts online, more needs to be known about the quality of those attempts and messages. Research on comforting communication and advice (MacGeorge et al., 2011), for example, offers guidance for evaluating the quality of support provision attempts online. The connection between support seeking and provision is another important topic to consider. Supportive communication is processual in nature. Understanding the relationship between specific support seeking behaviors and the types or quality of support elicited would be helpful. The role of communication technologies in constraining and enabling support provision also needs greater attention.

A final issue worthy of study in future scholarship concerns the support-related uses of communication technologies by patients within the context of their existing relationships with friends and family members. Online support sources tend to be studied as separate and distinct from offline sources of support such as family and friends. There is good reason to make such a distinction and continue to examine online support separately in future research. However, it is also critical to pay greater attention to how communication technologies are used for support within existing relationships. Important topics to consider include why and how patients use communication technologies to acquire support from family and friends. Blogs and social network sites, for example, may be a way to keep connected with more distant family and friends and, when necessary, more readily activate them as support resources. More broadly, it would also be valuable to further consider the interplay of online and offline support sources. The decision to seek support online is likely contingent on one's offline support resources. Further studying this topic would be a valuable direction for social support scholarship.

Conclusion

Several trends appear in research examining the implications of communication technologies for social support among people coping with illness. It is clear that various communication technologies are used by a significant number of U.S. adults to seek support from peers with similar health experiences. Substantial evidence suggests that settings such as online communities, blogs, and SNSs can be valuable resources for acquiring support, and the support perceived available in these contexts is associated with positive coping outcomes related to well-being. There is also good reason to believe that informational and emotional support are the most common types of support shared in online communities. Yet it is impossible to speculate about several other conclusions one might desire to draw. The consequences of support received online, implications of CMC for social support processes relative to face-to-face interaction, and the role of communication technologies in connecting with existing support resources available offline warrant considerably greater attention from scholars. Despite the progress made in this area, much remains to be learned to fully understand the support-related implications of communication technologies for digital coping.

4 Sharing Illness Experiences

Illness can be a profoundly disruptive experience (Bury, 1982). The series of physical, psychological, and social challenges that can accompany illness may interfere with the basic structures that define a patient's everyday life. Beyond creating uncertainty about taken-for-granted aspects of life, such as making breakfast or completing routine tasks at work, illness can raise fundamental questions about a patient's identity, place in the world, and future. The unique challenges presented by illness can create a need for patients to give voice to their experiences (Frank, 2013; Hydén, 1997). Indeed, sharing thoughts, feelings, and experiences can be a valuable means of coping with illness.

The thesis of this chapter is that communication technologies have important implications for how, why, and with what effects patients share their illness experiences. The chapter begins with an overview focusing on the role of narrative and self-expression in coping with illness along with a discussion of communication technology affordances relevant to this context. Motivations and content of online illness disclosures are next considered. The outcomes associated with sharing illness experiences online are then reviewed. The chapter concludes with an evaluation of issues that warrant additional attention in research on communication technologies and illness-related disclosure.

Illness and Self-Disclosure Background

To provide a foundation for this chapter, it is important to first consider some basic properties of illness-related disclosure. Accounting for one's condition and circumstances is an important component of coping with illness (Frank, 2013; Hydén, 1997). Narrative, which involves using traditional elements of stories to form an understanding of one's experiences (Sharf & Vanderford, 2003), can serve a number of different roles in the coping process (Arntson & Droge, 1987; Hydén, 1997). Perhaps most notably, narrative can aid in sense-making. Through retrospectively applying a structure to one's experiences, narrative makes it possible for those experiences to be better understood. It can also be a means for patients to assert control. Through creating an account and bringing order to their present condition, it is possible for patients to gain a greater sense of self-determination. A third function of narrative concerns transforming identity. Narrative provides an opportunity for patients to restructure their identity and incorporate or at least accommodate illness. Finally, narrative has a communal function that brings together people with common experiences.

Beyond narrative, the expressive writing paradigm (Pennebaker, 1997) plays a central role in research on illness-related disclosure. This paradigm is rooted in the assumption that writing about traumatic experiences such as illness can produce physical and psychological health benefits. As an intervention, expressive writing typically involves asking individuals to spend 15 to 30 minutes per day for between three and five days writing about a significant life event such as illness. Writers are encouraged to discuss their thoughts, feelings, and experiences with the event in detail. The broader benefits of expressive writing have been demonstrated in a plethora of studies. Several meta-analyses conducted to aggregate the results of expressive writing research have shown that expressive writing has positive effects on psychological well-being and physiological functioning (Smyth, 1998). Most notably, Frattaroli (2006) found that, across almost 150 studies, expressive writing was generally associated with beneficial outcomes (weighted mean $r = 0.075$). Another meta-analysis demonstrated the benefits of expressive writing specifically among people coping with one or more illnesses (Frisina, Borod, & Lepore, 2004). Research on expressive writing suggests that sharing illness experiences can be an important coping mechanism.

Self-Disclosure Affordances of Communication Technologies

Self-disclosure—which involves sharing information about oneself (Derlega, Metts, Petronio, & Margulis, 1993)—has been a topic of considerable interest among scholars studying communication technologies (e.g., Kim & Dindia, 2011; Ruppel et al., 2017; Suler, 2004). Several scholars have proposed that people may be more willing to self-disclose when using computer-mediated communication than interacting face to face (McKenna & Bargh, 2000; Walther, 1996). Suler (2004) illustrated this idea in discussing what he deemed an "online disinhibition effect" that occurs when "people say and do things in cyberspace in which they wouldn't ordinarily say and do in the face-to-face world" (p. 321). Yet the results of studies examining differences in disclosure between face-to-face and computer-mediated interactions have been mixed (Kim & Dindia, 2011; Nguyen, Bin, & Campbell, 2012; Ruppel et al., 2017).

Five affordances of communication technologies are particularly relevant to the context of discussing illness experiences. Control, anonymity, visibility, reach, and narrative potential considerations are addressed in the following paragraphs. Table 4.1 summarizes each of these affordances.

Compared with face-to-face interaction, some communication technologies offer increased control over the number or variety of social cues available to one's audience. In text-based interactions online, for example, patients' nonverbal behaviors such as eye contact and facial expressions are not visible to their audience. This control affordance allows individuals to dedicate greater attention to other aspects of the interaction such as message construction (Walther, 1996). Because less effort is required to manage nonverbal cues, individuals can better focus on what they are thinking and feeling. The control affordance may allow patients to better articulate their illness experiences.

Anonymity is a second affordance that has implications for self-disclosure among patients (McKenna & Bargh, 1998; Rains, 2014b; Tanis, 2008a, 2008b). Anonymity involves the ability of a communicator to conceal his

Table 4.1

Key Affordances of Communication Technologies Related to Self-Disclosure

Affordance	Definition
Control	Potential to manage aspects of interaction related to the types and amount of nonverbal behavior accessible to one's audience.
Anonymity	Potential to conceal one's identity.
Visibility	Degree to which one's behavior is observable by others.
Reach	Potential deliver a message to a particular audience.
Narrative potential	Potential to share one's experiences in depth.

or her identity (Anonymous, 1998). Although anonymity is often provided through features of technologies, the communicator's perception of anonymity is typically most important in determining his or her behavior. For example, one may use a pseudonym (e.g., JMK76) instead of one's legal name when communicating in an online support community but still not feel anonymous. Anonymity may reduce concerns about embarrassment or fears about retribution associated with sharing illness experiences.

The third and fourth sets of affordances that have implications for discussing illness are visibility and reach (Bazarova & Choi, 2014; Choi & Bazarova, 2015). Visibility involves the potential of others to see or hear one's messages. In blogging about illness, for example, a blogger's writing may be visible to a wide range of people, including friends and family members as well as unknown others. Reach involves the potential to share a disclosure with a particular audience, such as a specific person or community. One could send an e-mail to a specific individual or use a social network site (SNS) status update to broadcast a message to all or most of one's social network. The potential to reach a specific individual or the degree to which messages are observable to others may be used strategically by patients to foster different disclosure outcomes.

Narrative potential is a final affordance argued to have implications for self-disclosure online. It involves the degree to which a technology is conducive to sharing narratives (Merolli, Gray, & Martin-Sanchez, 2014). Narrative potential partially stems from the broader genre to which a communication technology belongs. Genre, which refers to the "socially recognized types of communicative actions [...] that are habitually enacted by members of a community to realize a particular social purpose" (Orlikowski & Yates, 1994, p. 542), is important because it implies how a technology should be perceived and used. Blogs, for example, are an extension of the personal journal genre (Herring, Scheidt, Wright, & Bonus, 2005). Belonging to this particular genre implies that the norms and practices common to personal journals should also be applied to health blogs (Rains & Keating, 2011). That is, blogging should consist of efforts to share one's innermost thoughts and feelings in a great deal of depth and without censoring one's self. Similarly, online support communities follow the genre of face-to-face support groups, where the expression of one's thoughts and feelings is encouraged. The narrative potential affordance allows patients to make more extensive illness disclosures.

Online Illness Disclosure Motivations and Content

With an understanding of some basic illness-disclosure properties and several technological affordances, it is important to consider why and how people use communication technologies to talk about illness. In the following section, motivations for sharing illness experiences online are first considered. The contents of illness disclosures in online settings are then discussed.

Motivations for Discussing Illness Online

Several motivations have been identified to explain why patients choose to share their illness experiences online. In one of the first studies examining this issue, Hardey (2002) evaluated 132 homepages authored by patients and found that they could be described by two dimensions involving patients' objectives and perceived expertise. Patients were motivated to explain their illness to others or provide support and viewed themselves as a novice or an expert about their health issue. These two dimensions were used to identify four different types of patient webpages. Homepages dedicated to the author's illness experiences largely consisted of narratives and served as a means of sense-making. Sharing experiences on a homepage helped to create a sense of coherence for the authors and had a therapeutic component. Homepages dedicated to serving as a source of advice were focused on producing and sharing health information. The goal of the author was less about the therapeutic benefits of talking about their experiences and more about using the knowledge they had gained to help others become more informed. The final two types of homepages discussed the author's personal experience with illness, but they did so in an effort to advocate for a specific solution (e.g., finding religion, alternative medicine) or promote a product (e.g., book) or service (e.g., pain institute).

Since Hardey's (2002) study, research examining motivations for illness disclosure online has tended to focus on blogging. Miller and Pole (2010) conducted an analysis of almost 1,000 health blogs and reported that more than 40 percent focused on the author's experience coping with illness. Yet they also found that more than 30 percent of blogs addressed health policy, business, or research, and half of all blogs were authored by health professionals. Other researchers have considered specific motivations for blogging about one's experience with mental health (Sundar, Edwards, Hu,

& Stavrositu, 2007), cancer (Chiu & Hsieh, 2013), and weight loss (Leggatt-Cook & Chamberlain, 2012). Throughout these studies, four motivations appear to be most prevalent. One major reason for sharing illness experiences online involves coping with the stressors presented by those experiences (Chiu & Hsieh, 2013; Chung & Kim, 2008; Ressler et al., 2012; Sundar et al., 2007; Yeshua-Katz & Martins, 2013). Writing about one's experiences can be cathartic and serve to relieve distress.

A second motivation for sharing health experiences in a blog involves connecting with others (Leggatt-Cook & Chamberlain, 2012; Ressler et al., 2012; Sundar et al., 2007; Yeshua-Katz & Martins, 2013). Discussing experiences served as a way for patients to overcome feelings of isolation and made it possible to form relationships and gain access to potential support providers. A third motivation concerns the desire to help others (Chiu & Hsieh, 2013; Chung & Kim, 2008; Ressler et al., 2012; Yeshua-Katz & Martins, 2013). Patients documented their experiences in an effort to assist others facing similar concerns. The fourth and final motivation is political in nature (Leggatt-Cook & Chamberlain, 2012; Sundar et al., 2007). Revealing the life of someone coping with mental health issues or obesity was a means for patients to correct misinformation and engage in social commentary about the ways these issues are viewed in society.

In addition to the four primary motivations pervasive across several studies, a few motivations for sharing illness experiences appeared less frequently but are nonetheless noteworthy. Among cancer bloggers, sharing one's experiences in a blog was done to prepare for death and leave something behind in order to be remembered (Chiu & Hsieh, 2013). Bloggers writing about their experiences with an eating disorder were motivated to cope with the stigma they felt (Yeshua-Katz & Martins, 2013). Finally, weight loss bloggers reported sharing their experiences to foster accountability (Leggatt-Cook & Chamberlain, 2012). The public nature of blogging effectively made them feel accountable for their goals and efforts.

A few limitations also may make patients reluctant to share illness experiences online. In interviews with bloggers writing about disordered eating, Yeshua-Katz and Martins (2013) identified several drawbacks, including being identified as having an eating disorder and triggering eating-disorder behavior. In research examining an online support community dedicated to Parkinson's disease, members were troubled by a lack of replies to their contributions, the inability to get to know other members beyond their illness, the departure of members from the community, and misunderstandings stemming from the lack of nonverbal cues such as facial expressions (Attard & Coulson, 2012).

Content of Online Illness Disclosures

A wide variety of content is disclosed by patients online. One theme in disclosure content involves technical issues related to illness and treatment. In mental health (Sundar et al., 2007) and cancer (S. Kim, 2009) blogs, breast cancer support communities (Chen, 2012a, 2012b; Høybye, Johansen, & Tjørnhøj-Thomsen, 2005; Sharf, 1997), and SNS groups dedicated to diabetes (Greene, Choudhry, Kilabuk, & Shrank, 2011), the discourse regularly focused on the classification of tumors, diagnoses, surgeries, medication side effects, or related medical issues. In one e-mail breast cancer support community, members discussed news stories about breast cancer and their challenges in dealing with physicians (Sharf, 1997). Illness-specific information was also identified in posts made about several different types of cancer by Japanese users of the microblogging service Twitter (Tsuya, Sugawara, Tanaka, & Narimatsu, 2014). Condition management was prevalent in discussions across breast cancer, type 1 diabetes, and fibromyalgia online support communities in another study (Chen, 2012a, 2012b).

Disclosure of technical issues related to illness extends to controversial topics and ideas counter to contemporary medical standards. An unproven medical therapy was the most widely discussed treatment by members of autism online communities (Zhang et al., 2017). However, community members were less likely to report actually using the therapy than accepted treatments. Disclosures reflecting misunderstanding and misuse were observed in a content analysis of posts made to the microblogging site Twitter about antibiotics (Scanfeld, Scanfeld, & Larson, 2010). Posts indicated a failure to understand the types of conditions for which antibiotics are appropriate and advocated the widely discouraged practice of sharing antibiotics. Researchers studying an HIV-denial community on an SNS identified several types of disclosures made by members related to technical aspects of the condition (Meylakhs, Rykov, Koltsova, & Koltsov, 2014). The scientific community was presented as lacking proof and antiretroviral treatment was framed as toxic.

A second theme in the content of patients' disclosures involves personal and emotional issues related to experiencing illness (Chen, 2012; Greene et al., 2011; Keim-Malpass & Steeves, 2012; Mulveen & Hepworth, 2006; Rodham, McCabe, & Blake, 2009). Exhaustion, fear, and loneliness were prevalent topics in contributions to an online breast cancer support community (Høybye et al., 2005). Patients in other online health communities reported resentment (Mirivel & Thombre, 2010), anger (Bar-Lev, 2008), and feeling misunderstood (Shigaki et al., 2008). In a study of mental health blogs authored by young adults, two core topics involved feelings of powerlessness and isolation (Marcus, Westra, Eastwood, & Barnes, 2012). Discussions of powerlessness were marked by patients' concerns about being oppressed by their mental health condition, feelings that it is all encompassing, and emotions such as fear and hopelessness. The loneliness theme was marked by feelings of an inability to connect, shame, and self-blame for one's isolation. Although negative emotions were pervasive, researchers also noted the presence of jokes and humor in a few studies (Marcus et al., 2012; Rodham et al., 2009). In one study, humor allowed online community members to talk about frightening or embarrassing topics and exert some control over their cancer-related condition (Demjén, 2016).

Other themes in disclosure content are less pervasive but still worth noting. Social support is one such theme identified in a few studies (Mulveen & Hepworth, 2006; Sharf, 1997). Online community members explicitly talked about the helpful support they had received by participating. Identity is another important theme. Discussions focused on what it means to be someone diagnosed with a specific condition such as diabetes (Greene et al., 2011) or a "good mother" (Kantrowitz-Gordon, 2013). A final theme involves the presence of commercial or promotional messages. Health-related advertisements were fairly common in the diabetes groups on the popular SNS Facebook (Greene et al., 2011) and cancer-prevention discourse was prevalent on cancer blogs (Kim, 2009).

Beyond general themes in the content of disclosures made by patients online, insights have been uncovered about disclosure structure and mechanics. In an analysis of 20 stories of cancer survivorship posted on the popular video-sharing website YouTube, almost all stories contained a diagnostic narrative detailing the survivor's experience being diagnosed (Chou, Hunt, Folkers, & Augustson, 2011). Most diagnoses were unexpected, and narratives involved depersonalized references to health care providers. Doctors and other medical personnel were rarely referred to by name and instead were described as "they" or "the doctor." Diagnosis narratives also typically included dramatic tension, marked by the inclusion of direct quotes about what the survivor said to his or her doctor and how the doctor responded.

Different types of disclosure structures were evident in other contexts. In one critical analysis of online communities for mothers coping with post-partum depression, disclosures were marked by confessionary language, language reflecting shame, and second-person accounts attempting to distance the author from her embarrassment (Kantrowitz-Gordon, 2013). Mothers gave several accounts for their depression, blaming themselves for not living up to their ideal of a "good mother," hormones or other physiological changes, or linked their depression to social dysfunction in their lives. These findings are consistent with another study in which most of the 30 stories from an online community examined by the authors highlighted the difficulties of postpartum depression, and almost half addressed concerns with failing to meet a perceived social standard for a "good mother" (Thomas, Scharp, & Paxman, 2014). Among people participating in pro-anorexia websites, communication structures included building a pro-anorexia identity, articulating self-loathing, advising others, and creating a sense of community (Haas, Irr, Jennings, & Wagner, 2011). These structures took the form of disclosures related to diet and exercise, discontent with one's body and self, tips and insights, as well as showing affection toward the community.

Stigma is a final topic that is relevant to patients' disclosure content. Stigma involves possessing a mark of discredit that is recognized by a particular social group (Goffman, 1963). It can limit illness-related disclosure (Greene, 2009) because patients coping with a stigmatized health condition may experience or fear social rejection (Fife & Wright, 2000) as well as threats to their physical safety (North & Rothenberg, 1993) or employment (Munir, Leka, & Griffiths, 2005). One researcher studying health bloggers found that, among bloggers who were more anonymous, those who experienced more illness-related embarrassment engaged in greater levels of self-disclosure (Rains, 2014). No such relationship existed among bloggers who were less anonymous.

Evidence suggests that responses to stigma-related disclosures are consequential. In one study, members of an online discussion community dedicated to concealable stigmas such as drug use were much more likely to make further contributions in response to receiving positive feedback to an initial post than members of groups dedicated to visible stigmas such as obesity or nonstigmatized issues such as cooking (McKenna & Bargh, 1998). Other researchers have further explored the content of responses to stigmatized disclosures in the context of a pro-anorexia online community (Chang & Bazarova, 2016). They found that when an initial post to the community contained stigma-related emotion words involving shame, anxiety, and embarrassment, negative emotion words were more likely to appear in the responses. The authors argued that negative emotion words validated the initial disclosure and reinforced the original discloser's negative feelings. Moreover, negative emotion words in response to an initial contribution increased the likelihood that further disclosures made by the original discloser would contain stigma-related emotion words.

Taken together, research examining the content of illness disclosures online suggests several conclusions. A few pervasive motivations appear to mark patients' decisions to discuss their illness experiences online. In addition to being motivated by a desire to relieve distress, patients disclosed their experiences as a means to connect with and help others. Limitations were also identified that might serve to undermine the desire to share illness experiences online. Patients' online disclosures appear to primarily concern two sets of issues. Patients discuss medical aspects of illness involving topics such as diagnosis, treatment, and care. A second set of issues involves the personal and emotional implications of coping with a health condition. A final conclusion that might be drawn from this body of research concerns the potential role of stigma. Although only a few studies have directly examined this issue, stigma may be important in what patients disclose online as well as their responses to positive and negative feedback from others.

Outcomes Associated with Sharing Illness Experiences Online

Having considered motivations for and content of illness-related disclosure, it is possible to evaluate the outcomes of sharing illness experiences online. Two primary topics have emerged in this body of research. The expressive writing paradigm has been applied as a formal intervention in several online settings. A second topic involves the effects associated with using specific forms of language in discussing illness experiences. These two topics will be considered in the following sections.

Expressive Writing Online

Several scholars have argued that writing online can be therapeutic and have drawn connections between writing and more traditional forms of therapy (Nagel & Anthony, 2009; Tan, 2008). Blogging, in particular, has been described as encouraging a kind of "personal translucence" in which the self is "put on view" in a "reflexive fashion, providing some kind of (admittedly distorted) mirror on the self, so that individuals might think about, reflect on, themselves and their everyday activities" (Graham, Rouncefield, & Satchell, 2009, p. 268). Others have focused on the cathartic potential of writing about stressors and claimed that writing may serve to make one feel empowered, relieved, and even exhilarated (Nagel & Anthony, 2009). Efforts to examine the effects of sharing illness experiences online tend to involve applying the expressive writing paradigm in this context.

Sheese, Brown, and Graziano (2004) conducted an experiment in which participants engaged in expressive writing about a traumatic or mundane event in their life via e-mail. Participants in the expressive writing condition tended to experience more positive health outcomes involving fewer sick days and symptoms of poor health than those who wrote about mundane life events. In another study, kidney transplant recipients were asked to engage in expressive writing about their transplant or discuss the medical facts related to the transplant (Possemato, Ouimette, & Geller, 2010). All writing was done on a secure website. Participants who wrote expressively experienced a greater increase in posttransplant quality of life than the factual writing group, but no difference was found between the groups in posttraumatic stress.

Other scholars conducted an intervention in which a group of women diagnosed with breast cancer received training on how to create and use a website that primarily consisted of a blog (Stanton, Thompson, Crespi, Link, & Waisman, 2013). Six months later, the results showed that the intervention was effective for women actively receiving breast cancer treatment. Participants in the wait-listed control condition who were receiving treatment experienced increased depression and decreased positive mood. In contrast, women in the intervention group who were receiving cancer treatment were no different from women not receiving treatment with regard to depression and positive mood. Taken together, all three of the preceding studies offer evidence that the effects of expressive writing extend to online settings. Yet none offers insights about how the unique aspects of such settings contribute to expressive writing outcomes—if at all.

The implications of engaging in expressive writing online were directly examined in one novel study. Boniel-Nissim and Barak (2013) examined the effects of writing publicly and receiving audience feedback. They randomly assigned a sample of adolescents experiencing social difficulties to one of several conditions in which the adolescents blogged about their experiences over the course of 10 weeks. All participants used a popular, publicly available blogging platform and were instructed to make two posts per week. Participants in the treatment group wrote about their thoughts and feelings concerning their personal relationships, and those in the control group were allowed to write about any subject they wished. The comments feature of the blog was also manipulated: half of the participants were able to receive comments on their blogs, and the other half had the comments feature disabled. A fifth group was included in which participants made entries in a personal diary kept privately on their computers as was a sixth group that did not engage in any writing.

Several noteworthy trends were observed in participants' changes in self-esteem, self-reported socioemotional difficulties, and participation in social activities. Participants who wrote about socioemotional difficulties and were able to receive comments, wrote about socioemotional difficulties with the comment feature disabled, and wrote about general topics with comments enabled tended to fair better than the group that engaged in general writing with comments disabled, the group who wrote in a private diary, and the group who did no writing. Experts also examined participants' writing to objectively evaluate their levels of socioemotional difficulties. Participants in the expressive writing conditions with and without the comment feature enabled experienced greater improvement than participants in the general writing/no comment condition.

Boniel-Nissim and Barak's (2013) study offers additional evidence that the beneficial effects of expressive writing extend to online settings. Writing about one's experience with a significant stressor online—whether via e-mail, blog, or in an online community—appears to produce at least some benefits to physical or psychological well-being. Perhaps more important, the results of their study also help to isolate some of the unique features of online settings that may influence the effects of expressive writing. One noteworthy difference between expressive writing online and traditional interventions is the nature of the audience. In traditional expressive writing interventions, writers are typically told that their writing is completely private (Pennebaker, 1997). In online settings, however, a patient's writing is likely to be public. Boniel-Nissim and Barak's (2013) study suggests that writing publicly may be beneficial. The expressive blogging groups with and without comments enabled experienced greater improvements in socioemotional difficulties and social activities than did participants who engaged in expressive writing using a private, computer-based journal.

Boniel-Nissim and Barak's (2013) study further suggests two specific mechanisms that may contribute to the effects of writing in public. The presence of an audience is one factor that appears consequential. The expressive blogging groups fared better than the group that wrote expressively in a private journal. Writing in a public domain may foster self-presentation concerns that encourage writers to frame their experiences more positively or less negatively than when writing alone. Public writers are more likely to worry about looking bad in the eyes of others when talking about stressful or potentially embarrassing experiences and privilege more positive or less negative interpretations of those experiences. Over time this may lead the writer to actually see those events in a more positive or less negative light.

A second mechanism that could make writing in public beneficial is audience feedback. Although Boniel-Nissim and Barak (2013) found no differences between the two groups that blogged expressively with and without comments enabled, it is noteworthy that these two groups also were not different from the group that blogged about general topics with the comment feature enabled. Additionally, the general blogging group that had comments enabled consistently fared better than the no-writing control group, but the general blogging group without comments did not. This set of results suggests that social interaction with blog readers may also be a benefit of writing in public. The feedback that participants received regarding their experiences may have been partially responsible for the benefits of expressive blogging.

Language Use in Discussing Illness Online

Beyond formal expressive writing interventions, specific types of disclosure content appear to have implications for patients' coping efforts and well-being. Much of this work has tended to focus on examining the effects of using specific categories of language when talking about illness on the discloser's coping efforts and well-being. Three categories of language have received the most attention: cognitive mechanism words, positive emotion words, and negative emotion words. Each category is drawn from the broader body of research on expressive writing and thought to reflect a different underlying coping mechanism (Pennebaker & Chung, 2007).

Insightful Disclosure and Cognitive Adaptation   One way in which disclosing traumatic life events such as illness may function is through fostering cognitive adaptation (Pennebaker, 1997). Articulating one's experiences in written form gives structure and helps to better understand those experiences. Cognitive mechanism words such as insight words (e.g., "realize," "understand") and cause words (e.g., "because," "reason") are two specific forms of language that serve as indicators that one is engaged in sense-making (Pennebaker, Chung, Ireland, Gonzales, & Booth, 2007; Pennebaker, Mayne, & Francis, 1997). These words are used to infer that a writer is making connections and engaging in self-reflection.

The use of cognitive mechanism words by patients participating in online communities has been linked with beneficial outcomes. In online support interventions dedicated to breast cancer, women who used more insight words reported decreased negative emotions and improved emotional well-being (Shaw, Hawkins, McTavish, Pingree, & Gustafson, 2006) as well as beneficial changes in health self-efficacy and functional well-being (Shim, Cappella, & Han, 2011). In a discussion community dedicated to the same topic, use of insight words was associated with increased functional well-being, decreased breast cancer concerns, and marginally improved physical well-being and depression (Lieberman, 2007). Yet other breast cancer research has been less consistent. Women who wrote a greater proportion of cognitive mechanism words (which includes cause and insight words) in one online support intervention reported increased emotional well-being, but use of these words was unrelated to changes in overall quality of life, health status, cancer-related intrusive thoughts, symptoms, or breast cancer concerns (Owen et al., 2005).

One possible explanation for the effect of using cognitive mechanism words among women coping with breast cancer involves a reduction in intrusive illness-related thoughts (Shim et al., 2011). Shim and colleagues found that the effects of insight words on health self-efficacy, emotional well-being, and functional well-being were mediated by breast cancer concerns. Their study offers evidence that insight words bring about positive effects among women coping with breast cancer by reducing their breast cancer concerns. Yet more research is needed to determine whether such effects are unique to women coping with breast cancer or would apply to other health conditions and groups. In a study comparing breast and prostate cancer online communities, for example, cause and insight words were marginally less prevalent in prostate cancer than breast cancer communities (Owen, Klapow, Roth, & Tucker, 2004).

Beyond online communities, some benefits of cognitive mechanism words have been observed among health bloggers. Hoyt and Pasupathi (2008) studied blogs authored by people who had experienced trauma and found that the use of cognitive mechanism words was marginally associated with recovery. Those bloggers who used more cognitive mechanism words experienced greater levels of recovery. In another study, the use of insight words by health bloggers was associated with decreased health-related uncertainty and, among those bloggers who wrote most frequently, increased perceptions of personal growth resulting from illness (Rains & Keating, 2015). Indirect evidence also highlights the importance of cognitive mechanism words. People who were pro-anorexia used significantly fewer cognitive mechanism words than did people recovering from anorexia in studies of personal homepages or discussion community posts (Lyons, Mehl, & Pennebaker, 2006) and blogs (Wolf, Theis, & Kordy, 2013).

Expressing Negative Emotions and Habituation   There is reason to believe that, under certain conditions, discussing negative emotions when sharing illness experiences online can be beneficial. Disclosing negative emotions is argued to encourage habituation (Pennebaker & Chung, 2007). That is, talking about negative experiences related to illness is a form of exposure that may, over time, lead to desensitization. As a result, those experiences have less of an aversive impact on one's coping efforts. Negative emotions are typically examined via the use of words that reflect a negative affective state such as "hurt" or "sad" (Pennebaker et al., 2007).

The results from research exploring the outcomes associated with expressing negative emotions about illness online have been fairly mixed. Among women with breast cancer participating in an online support intervention, use of negative emotion words was associated with increased breast cancer concern from baseline to intervention completion (Han et al., 2008). Women who expressed more negative emotions reported increased breast cancer concerns. Yet no connection was found between the use of negative emotion words and changes in health self-efficacy or emotional well-being among women with breast cancer in another intervention (Shim et al., 2011) or in health-related uncertainty among health bloggers (Rains & Keating, 2015).

The results from studies examining indirect outcomes of using negative emotion words have been no more consistent. Women who used more negative emotion words in describing their birth stories on a website were less likely to be involved in decisions made during the birthing process (Bylund, 2005). Yet people identified as recovering from anorexia used more anxiety words than pro-anorexics on their personal homepages or discussion community posts (Lyons et al., 2006) as well as their blogs (Wolf et al., 2013). Use of negative emotion words in initial posts made to an online cancer community increased the likelihood of a response in one study (Crook et al., 2015) but not in another project (Lewallen, Owen, Bantum, & Stanton, 2014).

The effects of discussing negative emotions appear to be nuanced and contingent on several factors. One factor involves how frequently negative emotion words are used. In an online support intervention dedicated to women with breast cancer, the authors reported an interaction between the volume of negative emotion words used during discussions and breast cancer concerns on changes in functional well-being (Shim et al., 2011). Whereas breast cancer concerns were associated with decreased functional well-being over the course of the intervention among women who used negative emotion words least frequently, they were unrelated to changes in functional well-being among women who used them most frequently. Participants only fared poorly when they used negative emotion words more infrequently. Rains and Keating (2015) reported commensurate findings in their study of health bloggers. Although negative emotion words were unrelated to changes in depression and perceptions of personal growth resulting from illness among bloggers who posted most frequently, use of these words was associated with increased depression and decreased perceptions of personal growth among bloggers who were least active. The findings from the two preceding studies suggest that infrequently expressing negative emotion might actually be detrimental. It could be that people who express negative emotion infrequently in coping with illness may not receive enough exposure to their aversive experiences to promote habituation.

Other research suggests that the effects of disclosing negative emotions are contingent on the degree to which positive emotions are expressed. In a study of bloggers recovering from trauma, those who experienced greater levels of recovery used a larger ratio of positive to negative words in their writing (Hoyt & Pasupathi, 2008). Yet at least some expression of negative emotion may be a necessary condition for benefitting from disclosing positive emotions. In an online support intervention, the use of positive emotion words was unrelated to changes in breast cancer concerns among women who wrote negative words relatively infrequently (Han et al., 2008). Among women who wrote negative emotion words most frequently, however, positive emotion words were associated with decreased breast cancer concerns over the course of the intervention.

Finally, there is reason to believe that expressing different types of negative emotions do not have the same effects. In two different studies, scholars have examined the expression of anger, anxiety, and sadness among women in online breast cancer support communities or interventions (Lieberman & Goldstein, 2006; Owen et al., 2005). Despite having similar samples, the results were fairly inconsistent. Expressing anxiety was associated with increased emotional well-being and reduced cancer-related intrusive thoughts (Owen et al., 2005) as well as with increased depression and decreased quality of life (Lieberman & Goldstein, 2006). Whereas the expression of sadness was not associated with changes in the two outcome variables examined by Lieberman and Goldstein (2006), it was associated with three of the six variables evaluated by Owen and colleagues (2005), including increased overall quality of life, emotional well-being, and decreased cancer-related intrusive thoughts. Expressing anger was not associated with any of the six outcome variables examined by Owen et al. (2005) and was only marginally associated with increased quality of life in Lieberman and Goldstein's (2006) study. One distinction between the two studies is that Lieberman and Goldstein (2006) evaluated these emotion words when they were used within 10 words involving cancer treatment. Owen et al. (2005) did not consider when negative emotion words were used by participants. However, that relatively minor difference would not seem to be responsible for such inconsistencies. Clearly, much remains to be learned about the coping outcomes associated with expressing particular negative emotions online.

Expressing Positive Emotions   Although the underlying mechanisms are less clear, discussing positive emotions related to one's illness experiences can be therapeutic. Lepore, Greenberg, Bruno, and Smyth (2002) claimed that "positive emotion can 'undo' or attenuate residual arousal and long-term distress that may result from negative emotional responses to stressors" (p. 103). Other researchers have drawn from Fredrickson's (2001) broaden-and-build theory to explain the benefits of expressing positive emotions. Positive emotions are proposed to broaden one's thought-action repertoire and bolster personal resources. Positive emotions encourage people to go beyond habitual modes of responding and think about the world and behave in beneficial ways. Interest, for example, is a positive emotion identified by Fredrickson (2001) that encourages exploration and may serve to expand the self. The expression of positive emotions has been typically examined via the use of words reflecting positive affective states such as "hope" or "happy" (Pennebaker et al., 2007).

Evidence for the benefits of discussing positive emotions online among people coping with illness is slim. Bylund (2005) reported that mothers who used more positive emotion words in their birthing stories posted online were more likely to be involved in decision making during labor. Yet other researchers have found no relationships between the discussion of positive emotions and changes in emotional or functional well-being (Shim et al., 2011) as well as cancer-related cognitions or breast cancer concerns (Owen et al., 2005) among women in online support interventions. Among health bloggers, use of positive emotion words was not associated with changes in depression or health uncertainty (Rains & Keating, 2015). Shim and colleagues (2011) even found that expressing positive emotions was associated with decreased health self-efficacy among the women in their research.

The findings from other studies have been no more encouraging or consistent. One group of scholars showed that people identified as being pro-anorexia used more positive emotion words than recovering anorexics in their personal homepage and online community postings (Lyons et al., 2006), whereas other researchers found no difference in positive emotion words on blog entries written by members of these two groups (Wolf et al., 2013). In studies of online support communities focused on cancer, the use of positive emotion words in an introductory post was associated with a greater (Lewallen et al., 2014) and smaller (Crook et al., 2015) likelihood of receiving a reply from other community members. Among microbloggers, posts about breast cancer that contained a greater number of positive emotion words were more likely to be forwarded or retweeted (Kim, Hou, Han, & Himelboim, 2016).

It may be that the expression of positive emotions needs to be considered in concert with negative emotions. Indeed, as previously discussed, positive emotion words have been shown to be associated with beneficial outcomes when the ratio of positive-to-negative emotion words is tipped in favor of positive emotions (Hoyt & Pasupathi, 2008) as well as among women who used negative emotion words relatively more frequently (Han et al., 2008). Contextual factors such as the nature of a health condition could also be important to consider. In one study, positive emotion words were used significantly more frequently in breast cancer online communities than prostate cancer communities (Owen et al., 2004). The type of positive self-disclosure was important in another study (Wang, Kraut, & Levine, 2015). Positive informational self-disclosure involving facts about one's experiences was associated with receiving more emotional support and less informational support. Positive emotional self-disclosures involving one's feelings, however, were not associated with either outcome.

Taken as a whole, several conclusions can be drawn from research examining the effects of using cognitive mechanism words, negative emotion words, and positive emotion words among patients online. One conclusion is that the way in which patients talk about their illness experiences online can be consequential. It is noteworthy that most of the intervention studies involved pretest-posttest designs, and each of these three classes of words were used to predict changes in patients' well-being after first accounting for their baseline levels of well-being. This is important because, although it does not definitively show a causal relationship, it does make it possible to be more confident that language use is at least partially responsible for the changes observed in well-being. Additionally, cognitive mechanism words, particularly insight words, most reliably predict improvements in well-being. Insight words had positive effects in several different contexts, such as online support interventions with a group discussion component, informal support communities, and health blogs. Sharing experiences in writing appears to be a particularly valuable approach for encouraging patients to make sense of those experiences and, as a result, cope more effectively. Finally, the effects of expressing positive and negative emotions are not well understood. One promising possibility is that the consequences of sharing positive and negative emotions are contingent on one another. That is, the degree to which patients benefit from articulating negative emotions may ultimately depend on the degree to which positive emotions associated with the event are also considered. An important challenge for researchers exploring this topic in the future is to better understand the optimal mix or conditions under which expressing both types of emotions produce the most beneficial outcomes.

Issues Warranting Greater Attention in Research Examining Illness Expression Online

A great deal of progress has been made in research examining the implications of communication technologies for sharing illness experiences. Despite this progress, several issues might be pursued in future research to further advance this body of scholarship. First, virtually every topic examined in this chapter is in need of additional research. Those factors motivating people to share illness experiences online as well as the content of such sharing merit further examination. More broadly, the connections among motivations for disclosing illness experiences online, the content of such sharing, and sharing outcomes deserve greater attention. It seems likely that these various components are interdependent. Patients' motivations for discussing health issues online may impact the nature of their disclosures and, ultimately, the outcome of those disclosures. Gaining insights about the entire process could help better understand each individual component.

Second, additional efforts are critical to better understand the role of communication technologies in patients' decisions to share illness experiences online and the outcomes of such disclosure. In a significant proportion of the research reviewed in this chapter, the implications of communication technologies were not fully considered. In several cases, online support communities, blogs, and SNSs appeared to simply be contexts in which to study other phenomena. Yet there is reason to believe that the social and technical characteristics that make these technologies unique—such as the affordances related to self-disclosure reviewed previously in this chapter—could influence the decision to disclose one's experiences as well as the nature and outcome of sharing. Advancing research on this topic demands isolating the implications of the communication medium for disclosure processes and outcomes.

Third, the collective nature of sharing illness experiences online deserves study. Moving beyond the individual, the shared discourse about experiences with an illness or a health condition is important to consider. In discussing online support communities, Davison, Pennebaker, and Dickerson (2000) noted that each individual participant's contributions served to create a "collective narrative that paints a portrait of identity by diagnosis" (p. 210). An opportunity exists to consider how a group's efforts in discussing illness serve as a collective form of coping. More broadly, it would be valuable to examine the ways in which illness is socially constructed through discussions occurring in various online contexts, such as online support communities and SNS groups.

Finally, it would be valuable to explore some of the negative outcomes or costs associated with sharing illness experiences online. This issue has only received scant attention to date, yet it seems reasonable to expect that there could be some deleterious outcomes of such disclosure. Issues related to privacy and privacy violations would be important to consider. It also seems possible that persistently discussing negative life events could encourage rumination or otherwise inhibit coping. The potential for unhelpful or even threatening feedback also warrants study. Examining issues such as these would help offer a more well-rounded view of the implications of discussing illness online.

Conclusion

Several conclusions might be inferred in reviewing the body of research examining the role of communication technologies in sharing illness experiences. A stable set of motivations appears to exist for discussing illness in online settings, including the desire to facilitate one's coping efforts. Expressive writing interventions can be successfully implemented online, and the use of cognitive mechanism words in discussing illness experiences plays an important role in physical and psychological improvements. Several other conclusions, however, are impossible to draw confidently. The implications of using positive and negative emotion words in sharing illness experiences are unclear, although their effects appear to be interdependent. The content typically present in illness narratives is not as well understood as might be desired. Perhaps most pressing, the uses and effects of those affordances that distinguish different technologies demand a great deal more attention from scholars. Efforts to examine these issues are critical to advance our understanding of when, how, and with what effects communication technologies are used to share illness experiences and, more broadly, their role in digital coping.

5 Seeking Health Information Online

Illness can provoke a significant number of questions. Patients may feel uncertain about the medical aspects of their diagnosis, treatment, or recovery. The psychosocial or financial challenges of illness can be a source of worry. Patients might wonder about the immediate and long-term consequences of their illness for their family. Information seeking is a critical mechanism for attempting to answer the bevy of questions that accompany illness (Johnson, 1997; Johnson & Case, 2012).

The central premise of this chapter is that communication technologies have important implications for the information-seeking behaviors of people coping with illness. The chapter begins with a discussion of some basic ideas about information seeking. Characteristics and motivations of patients who seek health information online will then be considered, followed by the mechanics of the information-seeking process. Issues related to information evaluation will be discussed next, along with the outcomes of seeking health information online. The chapter concludes with a discussion of issues that warrant additional attention in research on health information seeking.

Seeking Health Information Online

Health Information-Seeking Fundamentals

Prior to examining research on health information seeking online, it is first necessary to define key terms and identify some basic principles of information seeking. Information refers to "stimuli from a person's environment that contribute to his or her knowledge or beliefs" (Brashers, Goldsmith, & Hsieh, 2002, p. 259). It is a critical resource used to evaluate, maintain, or change one's health (Johnson, 1997; Johnson & Case, 2012). Information seeking refers to any intentional efforts to acquire information in response to a perceived gap in one's knowledge (Case, 2007). A key assumption of this chapter is that information seeking is an intentional act. Although some researchers have examined incidental or unintentional use of the Internet for health information (Shim, Kelly, & Hornik, 2006; Tian & Robinson, 2008a), it is assumed in this chapter that seekers are willfully trying to acquire information. Additionally, the Internet tends to be considered as a whole or single entity. It is important to note, however, that information seeking online may involve a range of activities from visiting a website to participating in online communities, social network sites (SNSs), blogs, or other activities (Lee, Hoti, Hughes, & Emmerton, 2014).

Three principles of health information seeking are particularly relevant to this chapter. First, information seeking is a process that may involve consulting several different sources. Health providers, family members, friends, newspapers, magazines, brochures, books, and several other sources may be used for health information. Indeed, numerous studies offer evidence that information seekers tend to consult multiple sources along with the Internet in an effort to acquire health information (Balka, Krueger, Holmes, & Stephen, 2010; Broom, 2005b; Ruppel & Rains, 2012). Although the role of the Internet will be privileged in this chapter, it is important to recognize that online sources of health information are typically embedded along with other offline sources during an information search.

A second principle of health information seeking is that a number of factors can influence the selection and use of an information source. Three classes of variables are outlined in the comprehensive model of information seeking (Johnson & Case, 2012; Johnson & Meischke, 1993). Demographic factors such as sex and education, health-related factors involving experience with a health condition, and source characteristics are all predicted to directly or indirectly influence source selection. Additional factors have been identified in other theories related to information seeking (Dutta-Bergman, 2006). Uncertainty, for instance, can lead information seekers to use or avoid an information source such as the Internet (Brashers et al., 2002).

Third, responses to acquired information can be complex. Although information may decrease uncertainty in some instances, it may serve to increase it in others (Brashers, 2001; Hogan & Brashers, 2009). Participants may feel more uncertain about their condition or prognosis. Acquiring information may also create a need for additional information. Information may inform one's coping efforts or be disregarded as patients choose to ignore the information they encounter. Responses to information acquired online can be nuanced, and it should not be assumed that obtaining information necessarily results in positive outcomes for the seeker.

Affordances of Communication Technologies Relevant to Information Seeking Online

In addition to discussing fundamental issues, it is important to consider the affordances of communication technologies that are particularly relevant to seeking health information online. Websites, online communities, blogs, SNSs, and related technologies can be distinguished from other health information sources in several important ways, including control, information diversity, availability, anonymity, and reach. Each of these affordances is summarized in table 5.1.

The affordance of control involves the potential for information seekers to manage the depth and breadth of a search (Rains, 2014). Relative to most other sources of health information, there are relatively few limits on the scope of information-seeking behavior online. Unlike acquiring information from a health provider where time and social protocol only allow a limited number of questions or a newspaper where one is limited to the articles presented in that day's paper, the extent of one's information-seeking efforts online are not subject to such restrictions. Information seekers may spend as much or little time and effort as they wish in searching the substantial volume of information available online.

Table 5.1
Key Affordances of Communication Technologies for Seeking Information

Affordance	Definition
Control	Potential to manage the depth and breadth of an information search.
Information diversity	Potential to access many different types of information.
Availability	Potential to acquire information when it is desired.
Anonymity	Potential to conceal one's identity when searching for information.
Reach	Potential to locate a specific information source or piece of information.

A second affordance for health information seeking involves the potential to access a diverse body of health information (Rains, 2014). Individuals may acquire technical information on webpages operated by reputable medical organizations (e.g., the National Institutes of Health) or medical journals, advice from medical professionals, stories shared by other patients coping with similar challenges, or several other types of information. The diversity of information available is important because it creates opportunities for seekers to meet their information needs. Relative to visiting a health provider who may not understand the day-to-day challenges experienced by patients or consulting family members who likely lack medical expertise, the diversity of information present online can make it possible for patients to meet their specific needs and address a range of health concerns.

Availability is a third affordance germane to health information seeking online. Unlike with a health provider, one need not schedule an appointment to acquire information online. It is possible to look for health information online any hour of the day or day of the year. The availability of health information makes it possible to acquire health information when it is most needed. As questions or concerns develop, anyone with Internet access can search online for answers. This affordance can be particularly critical for people who live in rural areas, lack transportation, or have impaired mobility.

The affordance of anonymity makes it possible to conceal one's identity—typically, one's legal name—when searching for health information (Ruppel & Rains, 2012). Health-related issues may be embarrassing or otherwise considered private. Searching for information can represent a risk because the information seeker may be forced to disclose his or her health status. Asking a friend for advice about a health issue, for example, also requires sharing that one is experiencing illness. Particularly when dealing with stigmatized health conditions, individuals may wish to acquire health information privately (Berger, Wagner, & Baker, 2005). The Internet offers several avenues for seeking information without revealing one's identity. Patients can avoid logging in to a search engine prior to browsing, use a pseudonym in online support communities, or several other means of concealing their identity while acquiring information.

Reach is a final affordance of communication technologies relevant to information seeking. Reach involves the potential to locate a specific information source or piece of information. One way that the Internet is unique as a health information resource is in the tremendous volume of health-related information present. This can be a benefit and a challenge to patients (Lee et al., 2014). Although sufficient answers to patients' questions may potentially exist, they might be difficult to locate. Reach centers on the degree to which patients perceive it possible to locate the particular information source or information that will meet their specific need. Relative to other sources, such as a health care provider or cable news, the Internet tends to allow for greater reach.

Information Seeker Characteristics and Motivations

Having provided background about health information seeking and communication technologies, it is now possible to discuss patients' information seeking online. This section explores who seeks health information online and the purposes for such efforts. In particular, the prevalence of information seeking online and the defining characteristics of information seekers will first be addressed. Common motivations for seeking health information online will then be examined.

Information Seeking Prevalence and the Demographics of Information Seekers

Researchers at the Pew Internet and American Life Project and the National Cancer Institute have conducted a number of surveys to better understand the health information-seeking behavior of U.S. adults since the year 2000. Their research offers evidence that Internet use to acquire health information is a pervasive phenomenon. Pew data showed that, during 2000, a little more than half of all adult U.S. Internet users sought health information online (Rice, 2006). By 2012, that number increased to 72 percent (Fox & Duggan, 2013). The results from the National Cancer Institute's Health Information National Trends Survey have been similar. The percentage of U.S. adult Internet users who looked for health information online during the previous year increased from 51 percent in 2003 to 79 percent during 2013 (National Cancer Institute, 2003, 2013). Beyond these two sources, several other large surveys have shown commensurate levels of health information seeking online by U.S. adults (Beaudoin & Hong,

2011) as well as adults in other countries such as France (Renahy, Parizot, & Chauvin, 2008).

Although the estimates are more variable than among the lay public, researchers have found that many people coping with illness use the Internet to acquire health information. More than 90 percent of patients with irritable bowel syndrome in one study reported having used the Internet to search for medical information (Halpert et al., 2007). In other research, more than three-quarters of patients eligible for bariatric surgery (Paolino et al., 2015) and sampled from one family medicine practice (Liszka, Steyer, & Hueston, 2006) sought health information online. Yet the prevalence of information seeking was lower in other studies. Among hematology outpatients in Belgium, half reported conducting a health information search online, and one-third indicated conducting a hematology-specific search during the previous year (Laurent, Cremers, Verhoef, & Dierickx, 2012). More than half of patients living with HIV/AIDS reported not having searched for information online since being diagnosed (Samal et al., 2011).

Several demographic characteristics distinguish online information seekers. Analyses of the lay public have tended to show that women (Beaudoin & Hong, 2011; Chisolm, 2010; Li, Theng, & Foo, 2015; Oh & Song, 2017; Percheski & Hargittai, 2011; Renahy et al., 2008; Rice, 2006) and people in poorer health (Chisolm, 2010; Li et al., 2015; Oh & Song, 2017; Powell & Clarke, 2006; Renahy et al., 2008; Rice, 2006) are more likely to seek health information online. However, exceptions to both trends have been reported (Powell & Clarke, 2006; Prestin, Vieux, & Chou, 2015). Education is another important factor, with people who have greater levels being more likely to seek health information online (Beaudoin & Hong, 2011; Li et al., 2015; Prestin et al., 2015). Although inconsistent findings have been reported in a few studies (Powell & Clarke, 2006; Rice, 2006), information seeking online appears to be more likely or prevalent among younger adults (Chisolm, 2010; Li et al., 2015; Prestin et al., 2015; Renahy et al., 2008; Tian & Robinson, 2008a). Several Internet-related factors can be consequential. People who used the Internet more extensively (Chisolm, 2010; Li et al., 2015; Renahy et al., 2008; Rice, 2006) or had greater Web-use skills (Dobransky & Hargittai, 2012; Percheski & Hargittai, 2011) or Internet self-efficacy (Lagoe & Atkin, 2015; Rains, 2008) were more likely to seek health information online.

Less is known about demographic factors that distinguish online information seeking among patients. In one study, patients with chronic illness who sought information online were more likely to be younger, have greater levels of education and income, and be in poorer health (Y. S. Oh & Cho, 2015). These findings are commensurate with the results of a survey conducted among hematology patients in Belgium in which patients who were younger and had attained greater education were more likely to have sought information for their condition online (Laurent et al., 2012). Illness- and coping-related factors also appear to be important. Among a sample of patients diagnosed with HIV/AIDS, people who sought information online had been diagnosed more recently and were more likely to have engaged in problem-focused coping (Kalichman et al., 2006).

Motivations for Seeking Health Information Online

Several motivations can drive online information seekers. At the most general level, information seeking has been described as being inextricably linked with coping. Adolescents experiencing chronic health issues, for example, reported feeling that information seeking was a taken-for-granted element of coping (Fergie, Hilton, & Hunt, 2016). They also felt that it was an important component of being a responsible patient. Several more specific motivations, which are adapted from Boot and Meijman (2010) and summarized in table 5.2, have been identified.

One widely cited motivation for seeking health information online involves the desire to acquire knowledge and, in particular, find and verify factual information (Boot & Meijman, 2010). In a study of young women

Table 5.2
Motivations for Seeking Health Information Online

Motivation	Definition
Acquiring knowledge	Desire to find and verify information related to one's health condition.
Managing uncertainty	Desire to cope with uncertainty related to one's health condition and increase one's sense of control.
Achieving solidarity	Desire to connect with others facing similar challenges.
Entertainment	Desire to pass the time or appease one's curiosity.
Accessibility	Potential to easily access large volumes of health information.

Source: The five motivations are adapted from Boot and Meijman (2010).

coping with breast cancer, for example, a primary reason for information seeking was to confirm their existing knowledge (Balka et al., 2010). German men with prostate cancer and women with breast cancer sought information online to become better informed about their situations (Kirschning & von Kardorff, 2008). The knowledge motivation extended to seeking information to prepare for or follow up after visiting a health provider (Colombo et al., 2014). Information seeking was even done to question health providers (Balka et al., 2010).

In addition to knowledge, a second and related motivation for information seeking online involves managing uncertainty (Boot & Meijman, 2010). This motivation is highlighted in research showing that information seeking allowed patients to gain a greater sense of control over their health condition (Balka et al., 2010; Kirschning & von Kardorff, 2008). Social motivations represent a third class of factors driving information seeking online (Boot & Meijman, 2010). Information seeking can be a means to achieve solidarity with others facing similar situations and may be more prevalent among patients who possess more meaningful social relationships. One study showed that people with a greater number of close confidants were more likely than those with few confidants to seek health information online (Askelson, Campo, & Carter, 2011). This finding, however, was not unique to seeking information online and extended to using other mediated and interpersonal sources for acquiring health information. Entertainment is a fourth motivation for seeking information online (Boot & Meijman, 2010). Information may be sought to pass the time. Researchers interviewing deaf adults reported that information seeking did not always meet an immediate need but was sometimes done out of curiosity (Karras & Rintamaki, 2012).

A fifth general motivation for seeking health information online concerns convenience. Patients use the Internet to seek information because it contains a variety of content, is easy to use, and is not limited by time (Choudhury, Morris, & White, 2014; Jones et al., 2014). Among oncology patients in Australia, the most common reasons cited for using the Internet included the convenience and availability of information (Newnham et al., 2006). These factors can be particularly critical for people who face health care barriers. Online information seekers in one study were more likely than those who did not seek health information online to report facing barriers to health care access such as the inability to get a timely appointment, reach a health provider via phone, visit a clinic when open, or have adequate transportation (Bhandari, Shi, & Jung, 2014). Convenience can also involve the potential to acquire technical information that has been translated for a lay audience (Kirschning & von Kardorff, 2008) and information available in one's native language (Yi & Zahn, 2010).

Beyond these five motivations, information seeking online appears to stem from more specific intrapersonal and situational factors. One particularly salient factor is health-related anxiety (Chae, 2015; Lagoe & Atkin, 2015). Relative to people low in health anxiety, researchers have found that people with higher levels of health anxiety searched for information more frequently online, spent more time searching, and experienced more distress from seeking information online (Muse, McManus, Leung, Meghreblian, & Williams, 2012). Some researchers have even posited the possibility of "cyberchondria," in which people who have high levels of health anxiety engage in information seeking online, which furthers their symptom-related concerns (Muse et al., 2012; Norr, Albanese, Oglesby, Allan, & Schmidt, 2015). In other words, Internet use serves to exacerbate initial health concerns and leads to more information seeking in an attempt to acquire reassurance. Other researchers have shown that greater perceived susceptibility to a mental health problem (McKinley & Ruppel, 2014) and lower levels of cancer fatalism (C. Lee & Chae, 2016) were associated with seeking health information online.

Stigma is another factor that can play a role in information seeking. In one study, respondents who self-reported a stigmatized health condition (e.g., depression, sexually transmitted infections) were more likely than respondents with a chronic condition that is not typically stigmatized (e.g., heart problems, diabetes) to have used the Internet to acquire health information (Berger et al., 2005). Respondents with a stigmatized condition were also more likely to report that using the Internet increased the number of times they visited a health care provider. Stigma is also associated with the use of specific communication technologies. In a study examining the content of search engine logs and posts to the microblog Twitter, moderate or highly stigmatized conditions were significantly more likely to appear in search logs than microblog posts (Choudhury et al., 2014). A final set of factors that may influence information seeking online involves environmental factors such as the media and public policy. Researchers examining the logs of popular search engines showed that legislation (Fazeli Dehkordy,

Carlos, Hall, & Dalton, 2014) and media coverage (Cooper, Mallon, Lead-better, Pollack, & Peipins, 2005; Fazeli Dehkordy et al., 2014) were associated with information seeking online. Searches for particular health issues were more common when they were the focus of legislation or received significant media coverage.

In discussing motivations for information seeking, it is important to consider information avoidance. Some patients may be motivated to actively avoid health information relevant to their condition. Deaf adults reported avoiding information seeking online in an effort to remain ignorant of information that could cause them to worry (Karras & Rintamaki, 2012). Avoidance was a strategy among young women facing cancer who felt overwhelmed by information (Balka et al., 2010) as well as patients with Lyme disease who did not want to encounter information that contradicted their explanatory model of the condition (Mankoff, Kuksenok, Kiesler, Rode, & Waldman, 2011). Parents of pediatric cancer patients reported initially refraining from seeking information online after their child was diagnosed (Gage & Panagakis, 2012). They were wary of what they might find and how that would make them feel. The fear of misinformation was also salient among this group. Although factors motivating information acquisition online have received much of the attention, the desire to avoid information appears to be a salient concern among some patients.

Taken together, the previously reviewed research indicates that use of the Internet for seeking health information is widespread—although its use specifically among patients appears to be more variable. People who seek health information online are more likely to be female, younger, more educated, and experiencing poorer health. Building knowledge is a primary motivation for information seeking. The convenience of information online and health anxiety are two other important factors. Information avoidance also appears to be an objective for some patients.

The Process of Seeking Health Information Online

Searching for health information can be a complex process. In this section, the topics examined by information seekers and mechanics of search behavior are considered along with the role of the Internet relative to other health information sources. This section concludes with a discussion of surrogate information seekers who search for health information online on behalf of patients.

Search Topics

Patients who use the Internet to acquire health information tend to search for one of two general topics. Technical information involves the medical aspects of a health condition, whereas experiential information focuses on the personal experiences of people coping with illness (Fergie et al., 2016; Kim, Shah, Namkoong, McTavish, & Gustafson, 2013). The key distinction between these two topics is whether factual information or first-hand accounts based on lived experiences with illness are privileged. Technical information is more likely to appear on health websites such as those operated by the Centers for Disease Control or the National Institutes of Health. Experiential information is more likely in contexts that privilege user-generated content such as online communities, blogs, and SNSs.

In searching for technical information, patients may attempt to acquire knowledge about their condition or its treatment. Men with prostate cancer and women with breast cancer reported seeking information online about diagnosis, disease trajectories, treatment, and long-term side effects (Kirschning & von Kardorff, 2008). Patients with multiple sclerosis indicated seeking information online for causes, treatment, and illness management (Colombo et al., 2014). Among patients with chronic illness, information about medicines and health providers was sought (Lee et al., 2014). Commensurate findings were reported in several other studies (Balka et al., 2010; Choudhury et al., 2014; Jones et al., 2014; Paolino et al., 2015).

Analyses of the logs created by search engines such as Yahoo! and Google provide additional insights about seeking technical information. These logs typically include records of queries submitted by individual users. In an analysis of 1.2 queries made to two commercial search engines during 2001, researchers reported that most searches were about topics related to technical aspects of general health, weight, reproductive issues, pregnancy, and personal relationships (Spink et al., 2004). In a three-month period during 2006, three of every 1,000 queries submitted to AOL's search engine addressed depression (Fu, Wong, & Yip, 2010). The two most common types of queries involved general topics related to depression or efforts to identify and manage depression. Google searches for status epilepticus made between 2004 and 2014 tended to address issues related to the definition, symptoms, and treatment of this condition (Brigo & Trinka, 2015). Users of the Mayo Clinic's website most commonly arrived at the website after searching for information about the symptoms, causes and treatment, or drugs related to one or more illnesses (Jadhav et al., 2014). These studies of search log data offer relatively objective evidence about the importance of acquiring technical information among patients.

Experiential information is a second general category of content involving how others cope with illness. Patients undergoing bariatric surgery reported seeking experiential information from other patients online to meet their psychosocial needs and for practical purposes such as determining how much time off work they would need (Paolino et al., 2015). Young women coping with breast cancer similarly wanted information unique to their circumstances as mothers and professionals with careers (Balka et al., 2010). Patients with multiple sclerosis looked for information about coping with everyday life (Colombo et al., 2014). As illustrated by these studies and other research (Laurent et al., 2012; Synnot et al., 2014), the purpose of information seeking was to acquire experiential information from others who were facing or had faced similar circumstances related to illness.

The types of information sought by patients depend on several factors. Culture can be important. In one study, participants from Korea and Hong Kong were more likely to trust and use sources providing experiential information such as blogs and SNSs than U.S. respondents (Song et al., 2016). U.S. respondents, in contrast, were more likely to use sources providing technical information such as WebMD.com. Another factor influencing the types of information sought is social support. Among women with breast cancer who had higher levels of emotional well-being, those who experienced low levels of social support were more likely than women who perceived higher levels of social support to search for experiential information and technical information related to breast cancer (Kim et al., 2013). Women lacking support engaged in greater information-seeking efforts. Treatment stage is another factor that can be influential. Among patients with fibromyalgia, information about dealing with pain was most important at onset and diagnosis, whereas information about treatment was more important after diagnosis (Chen, 2012a, 2012b). A final factor associated with the nature of information sought is the communication medium. Researchers reported differences in the types of medical information queried in search engines and posts made to the microblog Twitter (Choudhury et al., 2014). Whereas search engines were more likely to be used to acquire information about serious conditions, posts made to Twitter were more likely to address symptoms (e.g., tiredness, insomnia, irritation).

Search Mechanics

Several insights have been gleaned about the mechanics of patients' information-seeking efforts online. As opposed to starting at a specific webpage or health website, general search engines such as Google or Yahoo! tend to be the starting point for many searches (Karras & Rintamaki, 2012; Kuehn, 2013). Almost 80 percent of Internet users who participated in a Pew Internet and American Life Project survey indicated beginning health searches by using a search engine (Fox & Duggan, 2013). Data collected over the course of three months during 2005 from the website ClincicalTrials. gov showed that most referrals came from Google's search engine (L. Graham, Tse, & Keselman, 2006).

Despite consistent evidence about where many searches begin, less research has been conducted to examine the extensiveness of search efforts. Among oncology patients in Australia, more than half of online information seekers reported visiting four or more websites, and almost one-fifth visited more than 10 websites (Newnham et al., 2006). There also appear to be differences in search behavior based on the expertise of information seekers. In one study of search log data, medical experts used more complex queries and longer search sessions than members of the lay public (Palotti, Hanbury, Müller, & Kahn, 2016). Other researchers showed that the extensiveness of a search was contingent on how information seekers appraised the uncertainty they faced. In a laboratory study, participants who appraised uncertainty about skin cancer more as a danger and less as an opportunity conducted shallower searches in which they spent less time per webpage and visited more pages (Rains & Tukachinsky, 2015).

Patients may use one of several strategies when seeking health information online (Palotti et al., 2016). In one study, participants were randomly assigned to one of two scenarios involving a health concern and asked to search for information (Perez et al., 2015). All search behavior was recorded and evaluated. Three distinct online search behaviors were identified, including hypothesis testing, evidence gathering, and treatment/action seeking. Whereas hypothesis testing involved efforts to evaluate a diagnostic hypothesis about one's health issue (e.g., Do I have this particular condition?), evidence gathering focused on collecting information related to symptoms, and treatment/action seeking concerned looking for recommended courses of action. Related classes of search behavior have been reported by other researchers (Bulled, 2011).

Perez and colleagues (2015) used the three search behaviors they identified to catalog four broader search patterns. The first pattern, which was labeled a *simple search*, involved performing only one of the three search behaviors. *Intuitive searches* included two or more search behaviors and involved action/treatment seeking first followed by hypothesis testing or evidence gathering. The third search pattern, labeled an *analytical-recursive search*, involved at least two behaviors and began with hypothesis testing or evidence gathering but did not lead to action/treatment seeking. *Analytical-methodical* searches began with hypothesis testing or evidence gathering and led to action/treatment seeking. Notably, the researchers argued that simple and intuitive searches reflected shallower levels of attention to information content, whereas the two types of analytical searches reflected greater engagement with the content of information encountered during a search.

Other models of information seeking online focus on the process of information seeking as it unfolds over an extended period of time. At the most general level, a three-stage model was proposed that involved identifying a health condition, deciding whether to seek professional care, and accessing professional care (Bulled, 2011). In a study of patients with multiple sclerosis and their caregivers, information seeking was described as an evolving process (Synnot et al., 2014). Initially, several participants noted avoiding health information because they were wary of becoming unnecessarily fearful or developing false hope. Over time, however, respondents tended toward more focused and purposeful searches. The evolving nature of search behavior has also been documented by researchers studying search logs. One group of researchers found that, three weeks after an initial query indicating that the searcher had received care from a health professional, there was a spike in searches addressing benign explanations for symptoms (White & Horvitz, 2014). Searches for serious illness also increased after the first query reflecting care from a health professional.

In examining the mechanics of health information seeking online, it is important to consider barriers that make it more difficult. Several intrinsic and extrinsic barriers to information seeking were identified in a study of patients coping with chronic illness (Lee et al., 2014). Intrinsic barriers involved limited Internet literacy, lack of time and motivation, and questions about one's information needs. Extrinsic barriers included the availability of content (e.g., research journals), medical jargon, information inconsistency across sources, and the amount of information available. These intrinsic and extrinsic barriers served to mitigate information seeking online.

Internet as One of Many Information Sources

Researchers examining health information seeking online have tended to focus on the use and implications of the Internet in isolation of other potential information sources (e.g., health providers, friends, newspapers, magazines, etc.). Although good reasons exist for such an approach, evidence indicating that the Internet is one source among many used during health information seeking continues to accumulate. Among young women with breast cancer (Balka et al., 2010), deaf adults (Karras & Rintamaki, 2012), and other groups, the Internet was used in concert with several additional sources. In other research, the Internet was rated among the most important sources of health information along with health providers, family, and friends (Chen, 2012; Percheski & Hargittai, 2011). Evidence also indicates that information seekers' perceptions of other sources may impact Internet use. Respondents' trust in mass media and their health care provider was associated with their use of the Internet to acquire health information in one study (Rains, 2007b).

Channel complementarity theory offers one explanation for how and why multiple sources are used during a health information search (Dutta-Bergman, 2004, 2006). The central assumptions of this theory are that the Internet is one source among many, and source use is ultimately driven by engagement with an information topic. Sources—such as a health provider, family members, newspapers, magazines, and the Internet—are complementary to the degree that they serve the same function, such as providing health information. Channel complementarity theory predicts that patients who are motivated will consult all available sources that serve a particular function. For example, patients who are interested in learning more about a health condition such as prostate cancer will seek information online, from their family members and health providers, and from any other sources they believe will offer such information. Each of the different sources can potentially yield novel insights about prostate cancer. Researchers have found some evidence consistent with channel complementarity theory. In one study, Tian and Robinson (2008b) showed that people who sought information from their health care provider were more likely to attend to health information in newspapers, radio, magazines, television, and online.

An extension to channel complementarity theory has been proposed in an effort to make the theory more robust in the context of health information seeking. Although the degree to which sources are complementary has typically been discussed in terms of the specific types of content they provide (e.g., information about prostate cancer), researchers have argued that health information sources may also be used complementarily based on their characteristics (Rains & Ruppel, 2016; Ruppel & Rains, 2012). Four source characteristics were identified that, specifically in the context of health information, could serve as a basis for complementary source use: access to medical expertise, tailorability, anonymity, and convenience. Health information sources were proposed to be used systematically based on the degree to which they make it possible to access information from people who have formal medical training, offer information that is unique to the information seeker's circumstances, allow the information seeker to conceal his or her identity while acquiring information, and the relative difficulty associated with accessing and using a source to acquire information (Ruppel & Rains, 2012). Tests of this extension to channel complementarity theory demonstrated that sources were consistently used or not used by health information seekers based on the four complementarity characteristics (Rains & Ruppel, 2016; Ruppel & Rains, 2012).

Surrogate Information Seekers and Self-Quantification

Although much of the research conducted to examine health information seeking online tends to assume that seekers are acquiring information for themselves, people routinely seek health information on behalf of others. Data from the National Cancer Institute's Health Information National Trends Survey indicated that 46 percent of all U.S. adult Internet users sought health information online for someone else during 2003, 59 percent did so during 2005, and 68 percent served as surrogate seekers during 2013 (National Cancer Institute, 2003, 2005, 2013). Beyond their prevalence, comparatively little is known about surrogate information seekers and seeking. One group of researchers found that surrogate seekers tended to be younger and more likely to be married than people who sought information only for themselves (Cutrona et al., 2015). However, no differences were discovered between the two groups in perceptions of the effort required to search or problems encountered. More than half of the respondents to another survey indicated that they had volunteered to search for health information online on behalf of someone else, whereas one-quarter indicated being asked to conduct a search (Abrahamson, Fisher, Turner, Durrance, & Turner, 2008).

Parents are one important group of surrogate seekers. In a survey of parents visiting the emergency department of a hospital in Australia, more than 40 percent of respondents had searched for health information online for their children during the prior six months (Khoo, Bolt, Babl, Jury, & Goldman, 2008). Prior to their present visit, however, the Internet was only used by 6 percent of respondents. In a study of parents caring for an infant after a stay in the pediatric intensive care unit, mothers tended to be the primary information seekers (Kim, Garfield, & Lee, 2015). When searching for experiential information such as from blogs, mothers and fathers preferred sources that represented their unique perspectives. In another study examining parents of newborns, the Internet was used in response to their unfamiliarity with medical jargon, unpredictability of events, emotions related to uncertainty, and feelings of anxiety. Parents who expected to find positive or reassuring information were more likely to actively search for information, whereas those expecting negative or concerning information only searched when they felt capable of dealing with the results. In other research, parents of children with cancer similarly reported that the Internet was useful for particular types of information such as clarifying medical terms and instructions from health providers (Gage & Panagakis, 2012).

Information-seeking efforts also extend to collecting and procuring one's own health data. Efforts at self-quantification, which have been referred to as personal analytics, involve using technologies to track and monitor data about one's health (Almalki, Gray, & Martin-Sanchez, 2016). A range of health behaviors may be tracked, including physical activity, food, sleep, and weight (Choe, Lee, Lee, Pratt, & Kientz, 2014). Some principle motivations for tracking include entertainment, self-discipline, health, self-optimization, and associating with others (Gimpel, Nißen, & Gorlitz, 2013). Notably, a connection appears to exist between what is being tracked and motivations for tracking. Self-discipline motivation was positively associated with tracking physical activity and nutrition information in one study, whereas entertainment was correlated with tracking things in one's environment and the desire to associate with others was correlated with tracking addiction behaviors (Gimpel et al., 2013). The potential to associate and compare oneself with others has also been shown to influence health beliefs in the context of self-quantification. Relative to only receiving self-tracking feedback about their own exercise, participants in one experiment who also received feedback about others' performance reported feeling more health conscious (Gimpel et al., 2013). Although research on this topic is just beginning, self-quantification activities appear to have several possible health implications.

Several noteworthy trends exist in research examining the process of seeking health information online. Two broad classes of information are most sought, including information about technical aspects of illness and experiential information involving others' experiences with a health condition. Evidence suggests that information seeking is an evolving process marked by specific behaviors and broader classes of search strategies. Researchers have also begun to better understand how the Internet is used in combination with other sources in acquiring health information. Source complementarity characteristics appear to play an important role in source use during the health information-seeking process. Finally, significant numbers of U.S. adults serve as surrogate seekers who search for health information online on behalf of someone else.

Information Evaluation and Search Outcomes

Beyond the search process, several nuances of seeking health information online are important to consider. One topic involves how information seekers evaluate the health information they encounter. Another issue concerns the outcomes of information seeking for patients' physical health and psychosocial well-being. Both of these topics will be considered in the following sections.

Evaluating Online Health Information

A paradox appears to exist involving information seekers' perceptions and use of the Internet as a source for health information. One consistent finding across numerous studies involving a range of health issues has been that at least some patients had significant concerns about the quality of health information available online. For example, almost one-fifth of patients undergoing bariatric surgery reported feeling that the surgery-related information available online was untrustworthy (Paolino et al., 2015). In focus groups among people facing multiple sclerosis, several respondents indicated being wary of online health information (Colombo et al., 2014). Research conducted among adults with hearing loss (Karras & Rintamaki, 2012) and women with breast cancer (Balka et al., 2010) offered further evidence of skepticism about the quality of online health information. Despite such concerns, however, the usage statistics discussed previously in this chapter offer evidence that the Internet has been a widely used health information resource. Patients consistently register concerns with information quality but nonetheless continue to seek health information online.

There is also reason to believe that the magnitude of concern with information quality may not be proportional to the threat. Although only a few studies have been conducted, research examining the quality of health information available online in contexts such as discussion communities has tended to show that misinformation was not pervasive. In an analysis of more than 4,000 posts made to a breast cancer online community, 10 posts were identified by medical professionals as containing false or misleading information (Esquivel, Meric-Bernstam, & Bernstam, 2006). Moreover, 7 of the 10 were eventually identified and corrected by other members of the discussion community. Researchers analyzing 25 discussion threads addressing HIV, diabetes, or chickenpox posted among three websites found that health information was more likely than not to contain high-quality information by a factor of 4 to 1 (Cole, Watkins, & Kleine, 2016). The lowest possible rating was only awarded 3 percent of the time, whereas the highest rating was awarded in 15 percent of evaluations. These results can be contrasted with the findings from an analysis of 100 websites addressing common pediatric conditions and targeted to children (McPherson, Gofine, & Stinson, 2014). On average, these websites only received a moderate quality rating. However, there was a great deal of variability in ratings and the rating tool had poor test-retest reliability.

Related to information quality, preliminary evidence suggests that online communities and community members recognize the limits of their expertise and the importance of medical professionals. In an analysis of 1,700 threads from a diabetes community on the website WebMD.com, one researcher found 39 threads in which patients were instructed by a moderator to consult with their doctor instead of the community (Huh, 2015). These instances occurred when a community member posed a clinical question. In almost half, the moderator's instructions led to no further contributions—from the initiator or other members—to the thread. Most of the patients who were told to visit a doctor did not make any other contributions to the community, but this trend was not different from broader participation patterns in the community.

Other research indicates that patients may not be careful consumers of online health information. In one study, patients coping with HIV/AIDS were asked to evaluate a webpage containing high-quality information about the topic from a reputable source (i.e., *Journal of the American Medical Association*) and a second webpage with low-quality information from a questionable source (Kalichman et al., 2006). Although the low-quality webpage was rated less positively than the high-quality page, participants nonetheless viewed the low-quality page favorably. Further, participants with an avoidant coping style were more likely to positively evaluate the low-quality webpage. Other research underscores information seekers' difficulties evaluating health information online. In one study, participants were randomly assigned to read a message on a health website authored by "Anonymous" or "Pat Thomas" (Rains, 2007a). Although contemporary guidelines for acquiring health information online routinely include recommendations about being wary of anonymous sources (e.g., MedlinePlus, 2015), no differences were found in the perceived credibility or influence of the anonymous and identified sources. Researchers have also uncovered biases in search behaviors. One such bias involves only attempting to locate confirming information when evaluating the validity of a claim (Kayhan, 2013). This bias leads information seekers to fail to consider contradictory evidence, which is critical for rigorously evaluating a claim.

One theoretical explanation about how people evaluate the quality of health information they encounter online can be found in the MAIN model (Sundar, 2008). In this model, cues available in online contexts serve to trigger heuristics used in evaluating sources and information. Heuristics are simple decision rules that can be applied in evaluating sources and information. One heuristic that might be triggered online is the rule that information from experts tends to be correct. Four sources of cues are identified in the MAIN model that can trigger heuristics, including modality, agency, interactivity, and navigability. Modality involves how information is presented (e.g., text, audio, audiovisual), whereas agency reflects the presumed source of the information (e.g., a specific reporter, website, other site users). Interactivity stems from the potential to directly engage an information source (e.g., entering information into a website and receiving individualized feedback). Navigability involves moving from one location to the next (e.g., using a hyperlink and moving to another part of a website). These four types of cues can encourage information seekers to apply one or more particular heuristics in evaluating the quality of health information they encounter.

An experiment conducted to examine perceptions of credibility related to online health information and sources illustrates the role of agency in source evaluations. Hu and Sundar (2010) randomly assigned their participants to read and evaluate the same health message ostensibly posted to a website, online community, blog, or personal homepage, or simply attributed to "the Internet." Participants who read the information on a website reported being significantly more likely to follow or share the advocated advice than when the message was on a blog, homepage, or "the Internet." More important, the impact of the source (i.e., website, blog, etc.) on participants' intentions to adopt or share the advice was mediated by their perceptions that the source was controlled by professional editors or other users. Consistent with the MAIN model (Sundar, 2008), the context in which the information was presented triggered a heuristic about the presence of gatekeepers monitoring the quality of information online. This heuristic ultimately impacted participants' responses to the health message—in this case, leading the exact same information to be more influential when presented on a website than in other contexts.

Beyond the MAIN model, researchers have sought to better understand strategies used to evaluate health information and sources. In focus groups, undergraduate students reported using different criteria to evaluate the credibility of health websites and messages (Prybutok & Ryan, 2015). Whereas health messages were evaluated using the presence of statistics, references, and specific information as well as their consistency with participants' prior experience and knowledge, factors such as name recognition and good reviews from others were also used to assess website credibility. Other researchers have found a connection between the number of structural features included in a health website such as third-party endorsements, links to external websites, and a privacy policy statement and perceptions of site credibility (Rains & Karmikel, 2009). Verifying information across multiple sources—including with health professionals (Paolino et al., 2015)—was another information evaluation strategy used by adolescents coping with chronic illness (Fergie et al., 2016) and people facing Lyme disease (Mankoff et al., 2011).

Intrapersonal factors related to health literacy appear to play an important role in determining the rigor of information evaluation efforts. A systematic review indicated that people with lower health literacy were less able to evaluate health information online and had lower levels of trust in online information (Diviani, van den Putte, Giani, & van Weert, 2015). Other researchers found that pregnant women with lower health literacy were less likely to seek information online than women with higher health literacy (Shieh, Mays, McDaniel, & Yu, 2009). However, no differences were found between the two groups in their use of traditional media or interpersonal sources of health information. Health literacy was also associated with health information seeking online in studies of adolescents (Ghaddar, Valerio, Garcia, & Hansen, 2012) and low-income adults (Jensen, King, Davis, & Guntzviller, 2010).

The Outcomes of Seeking Information Online
The consequences of seeking health information online for physical health and psychosocial well-being are important to discuss. Although it has received relatively less attention than other issues, some evidence suggests that information seeking online may be associated with positive outcomes. In a survey of patients with irritable bowel syndrome, respondents who had sought health information online were more informed about the condition and generally had fewer misconceptions relative to respondents who did not search for information online (Halpert et al., 2007). Among a sample of HIV/AIDS patients, online information seeking was positively associated with antiretroviral therapy adherence (Samal et al., 2011). Other research has shown that information seeking online may be particularly useful for managing uncertainty about cancer prevention (Rains, 2014). Relative to

people who did not seek cancer information, online information seekers' actual level of uncertainty about cancer prevention was more aligned with the level of uncertainty they desired.

Perhaps the most compelling evidence of the benefits stemming from information seeking online can be found in a longitudinal study of people with inflammatory bowel disease that was conducted over seven months (Sassenberg & Greving, 2016). The researchers proposed that Internet use would be a means for patients who experienced frequent illness episodes to gain a more positive perspective about their health. They found an interaction between the frequency of acute illness episodes and online information seeking for health changes evaluated in terms of health-related stress, self-esteem, and risk perceptions. Among people who sought information more frequently, increased episodes of illness were associated with improved health. This relationship was not observed among people who sought information less frequently. Moreover, the relationship between illness episodes and changes in health was not impacted by offline information seeking or online support community use. The results from this study indicate that information seeking can be a particularly valuable mechanism for coping with illness. Information seeking can be used to help better understand and manage episodes of acute illness.

Other researchers have reported more mixed or even negative consequences of seeking health information online. In a survey of older adults in The Netherlands, for example, more than one third of the sample reported that health information seeking online sometimes or often helped them to make lifestyle changes as well as question a diagnosis or treatment (Medlock et al., 2013). Internet use also made respondents feel reassured and knowledgeable but also anxious and confused. Among hematology patients in Belgium, positive outcomes such as finding background information and feeling reassured were identified along with negative outcomes such as increased worry and encountering inaccurate or poor quality information (Laurent et al., 2012).

Several researchers have focused specifically on the implications of information seeking online for health-related anxiety. In a longitudinal study, seeking cancer information from online news was associated with increased worry of developing cancer (Chae, 2015). Notably, the effects stemming from consumption of online news were not observed with other sources of information online. Seeking cancer information from professional health-related websites or using SNSs was not associated with changes in cancer worry. Other researchers found that health anxiety moderated the relationship between online health information seeking and visiting a health provider (Eastin & Guinsler, 2006). Among people with moderate and high levels of health anxiety, online information seeking was associated with a greater likelihood of visiting a doctor.

To summarize, research examining the nuances of health information seeking online offers several insights about how information is evaluated and the outcomes of information seeking. A paradox appears to exist in which, despite being wary of information quality, the Internet is routinely used for seeking health information. This paradox is particularly noteworthy given research indicating a lack of widespread misinformation online and deficits in seekers' information evaluation skills. Examining the role of decision heuristics triggered by contextual cues is one promising avenue for better understanding how patients evaluate health information online. Relatively little research has been conducted to evaluate the outcomes of seeking health information online, and the results of existing studies are mixed. Although some tentative evidence suggests that information seeking can be beneficial, those studies demonstrating deleterious outcomes cannot be ignored.

Issues Warranting Greater Attention in Online Health Information-Seeking Research

The research reviewed in this chapter underscores the important implications of seeking health information online among patients. Despite the significant contributions made by existing research, several issues merit additional attention. First, a relatively substantial amount is known about the use of the Internet to acquire health information by the general population of U.S. adults. Beyond the prevalence of such behavior, a clear pattern of demographic characteristics distinguish people who are more and less likely to seek health information online. One important issue that deserves further consideration is the prevalence and demographic factors that distinguish online information seeking specifically among patients. Better understanding the implications of online information seeking among this group requires first determining who is more and less likely to engage in this behavior.

A second issue meriting greater attention involves the reasons for and consequences of seeking specific types of health information. When and why, for example, is technical and experiential information sought by people coping with illness? How do these two different classes of information impact coping efforts? More broadly, it is essential to further examine the mechanics of information seeking. Researchers need to know more about the strategies people undertake in seeking health information online. Although the few existing studies offer important insights, additional efforts are necessary to more fully understand what patients do in attempting to acquire health information online.

Third, it is critical to more fully consider the role of the Internet in broader information-seeking efforts. As was noted at several points in this chapter, the Internet is one source among many that may be used to acquire health information. It is critical to further investigate Internet use in concert with other sources. Moreover, it is important to move toward examining the Internet not as a whole but as a collection of individuals sources (e.g., online communities, websites, SNSs, etc.). The affordances outlined in this chapter offer a starting point to begin thinking about the Internet in more nuanced ways.

A final issue deserving greater attention in research on health information seeking online concerns information-seeking outcomes. Relatively little research has been conducted to explore how information seeking online impacts patients' coping efforts. It is critical to examine more immediate outcomes, such as responding to specific concerns, as well as long-term consequences like recovery time or relapse. Focusing on the outcomes of information seeking and factors that contribute to more and less positive outcomes is particularly essential for developing strategies that could be employed by health care professionals to assist patients. It seems reasonable that some basic principles could be developed that would help patients capitalize on information seeking to more effectively cope with illness—or at least avoid the major pitfalls of acquiring health information online.

Conclusion

Several conclusions can be drawn from research examining health information seeking online among patients. Health information seeking among U.S. adults is widespread. The primary motivations for seeking health information online stem from the desire to accrue knowledge about a health condition and the accessibility of information. Although relatively little research has been conducted to examine the mechanics of information seeking, substantial evidence indicates that information seekers attempt to acquire technical information about an illness as well as experiential information from others facing similar circumstances. The quality of health information available online is a persistent concern for information seekers, despite little evidence that misinformation is pervasive. Tentative evidence suggests that information seeking can be beneficial, but researchers have also reported no or even negative outcomes in the form of confusion and anxiety. As with many of the topics addressed in this book, additional research is essential to further explore each of the preceding issues. Such efforts are critical to develop a more robust understanding of the implications of communication technologies for acquiring health information and coping with illness digitally.

6 Changing Patient-Provider Relationships

Health care providers can play an integral role in patients' efforts to cope with illness (Roter & Hall, 2006). Primary care physicians, medical specialists, nurses, and other health providers can be critical resources for information, care, and support. The connections between patient-provider relations and patients' health outcomes have been documented in numerous empirical studies (Brown, Stewart, & Ryan, 2003; Duggan & Thompson, 2011). Some patients, however, may experience significant difficulties in communicating with their health care provider. Beyond basic misunderstandings such as confusion over treatment instructions, more fundamental problems may exist stemming from the assumptions that these two groups make about one another's roles. A central challenge for researchers has been to understand the conditions under which the patient-provider relationship is beneficial and problematic for patients' coping efforts.

The thesis of this chapter is that communication technologies have significant implications for patient-provider communication and relationships. After first providing background information about patient-provider relations and the affordances of communication technologies relevant to these two groups, patients' Internet use will be considered. The role of health information from the Internet during medical consultations is next discussed. The uses and effects of e-mail as a communication tool for patients and health providers are then examined, followed by a discussion of social media and health providers. The chapter concludes with a review of issues warranting greater attention in research on patient-provider relations and communication technologies.

The Patient-Provider Relationship

Fundamentals of Patient-Provider Communication

Before considering the implications of communication technologies, it is first important to discuss some basic properties of patient-provider communication. The relationship between a given patient and health provider can be distinguished on several dimensions. One important distinction involves the level of control over decision making perceived and desired by patients and providers (Emanuel & Emanuel, 1992; Roter & McNeilis, 2003). A paternalistic relationship occurs when providers have a high level of control and patients' control is low. Providers function as a guardian for patients and, given their advanced training, make decisions on behalf of patients. A consumerist relationship occurs when patient control is high and provider control is low. In these relationships, patients take sole responsibility for their decision, and providers are relegated to serving as one information source and a technical expert. A mutual relationship involves both patients and providers having high levels of control. In these relationships, decision making and care become a collaborative endeavor, and the provider acts as an advisor. The final type of relationship occurs when both patients and providers have low levels of control. These deficient relationships are marked by a great deal of uncertainty and disharmony.

A general shift appears to be occurring in the roles of patients and health providers away from the paternalistic model and toward greater patient involvement and control. One hallmark of this shift has been an increased focus on patient-centered communication (Stewart et al., 2000). Although it has several different dimensions, patient-centered communication involves understanding the patient's perspective, achieving shared understanding, and encouraging patient involvement (to the degree that he or she is comfortable) (Epstein et al., 2005). These ideas are also prevalent in research on collaborative decision making, in which patients play an active role and providers attempt to achieve a shared understanding and cooperatively mange uncertainty (Charles, Gafni, & Whelan, 1997; Politi & Street, 2011). Other researchers have made broader arguments about patient empowerment, in which the traditional power dynamic between patients and providers is redistributed and patients become more actively involved in their own health care (K. J. Roberts, 1999). The availability of medical information on the Internet is particularly critical in creating opportunities for empowerment. Medical professionals have less of a monopoly on health information, and patients have a means to gain expertise about health issues as well as become health information producers (Broom, 2005b; Hardey, 2001). The efforts of patients to take an active role in their care will be an important issue among several of the topics addressed in this chapter.

Affordances of Communication Technologies Relevant to Patients and Providers

In addition to offering background information about patient-provider communication, it is important to consider the unique affordances of communication technologies that are particularly relevant to these two groups. Although communication technology use among patients and providers dates back to at least the telephone during the late 1800s (Spielberg, 1998), this topic did not receive significant attention until relatively recently. Researchers began to consider the implications of telemedicine (Field, 1996) and e-mail (Baur, 2000; Spielberg, 1998) for patient-provider communication. Across these older technologies as well as contemporary forms of social media such as blogs and social network sites (SNSs), four affordances are particularly relevant: information diversity, availability, documentation, and visibility. Each affordance represents a way that communication technologies are perceived or used by patients and providers to interact with one another or otherwise has important implications for the patient-provider relations. The four affordances are summarized in table 6.1.

Communication technologies provide a great deal of access to both formal and informal sources of medical information. This information

Table 6.1
Key Affordances of Communication Technologies for Patients and Providers

Affordance	Definition
Information diversity	Potential for patients and providers to acquire or produce different types of medical information.
Availability	Potential to access a patient or provider outside of traditional medical consultations.
Documentation	Potential to have a written record of an interaction between patients and providers.
Visibility	Potential to become aware of others' presence or behavior.

diversity affordance is important because, as previously discussed, medical professionals have traditionally had a monopoly on health information (Broom, 2005b; Hardey, 1999). For patients, the Internet can serve as an alternative information source. Patients can find formal medical or clinical information about diagnoses and treatments as well as information about others' lived experiences with a health condition. Information diversity also extends to the opportunity for patients to become producers of medical information. Patients can share what they have learned or experienced on a blog, online community, or other context. For health providers, technologies such as blogs offer a means to acquire information about the everyday lives of people coping with a particular health condition.

Availability is a second affordance of communication technologies relevant to patient-provider interaction. Availability involves the possibility of contacting one another outside of a traditional medical consultation. E-mail, in particular, has been heralded for its potential to increase opportunities for interaction among patients and providers (Baur, 2000; Spielberg, 1998). Particularly given the relatively short period of time spent together during office visits, e-mail is a means for patients to share information that might be helpful in their care. These increased interactions may serve to bolster the connection between patients and providers and ultimately benefit both parties. Providers can better understand their patients; as a result, patients receive care that best meets their needs.

A third affordance of communication technologies important for patient-provider relations is documentation. Although e-mail is most notable in this regard, several communication technologies make it possible to produce a written record of interactions between patients and providers. For health providers, such documentation can function to enrich a patient's medical file (Spielberg, 1998). Providers can have a more complete account of their discussions with patients. Documentation can also be important for patients. Having a written record allows patients to better understand their health history as well as specific recommendations made by a provider.

Visibility is a final affordance of communication technologies relevant to patients and health providers. Visibility involves being able to observe or become aware of others' presence or behavior. At the most basic level, communication technologies make it possible for patients and providers to remind one another of their relationship and reinforce their connection.

For patients, the act of sending an e-mail message may go well beyond the specific issue addressed and serve as a means to remind providers of their continued need for assistance. An e-mail response may allow providers to demonstrate to patients that they are concerned and dedicated. Providers may also use a practice website or SNS page to make known or reinforce their presence among current and prospective patients.

Internet Use and the Patient-Provider Relationship

With the previous background information in place, it is now possible to evaluate research exploring the role of communication technologies in patient-provider communication and relationships. Patients' Internet use is connected to the patient-provider relationship in several ways. First, the quality of patients' relationships with their providers contributes to patients' use of the Internet to acquire medical information (Hou & Shim, 2010; Kivits, 2006; Song, West, Lundy, & Dahmen, 2012; Tustin, 2010). Patients who evaluate their health provider as less person-centered or are unhappy with the information they receive are more likely to search for health information online.

In a study of patients recruited from health provider offices, those patients who reported spending more time searching online for information about a health problem were less satisfied with the amount of time they spent with their provider and felt that their provider knew them less well (Tanis, Hartmann, & te Poel, 2016). Similarly, members of a cancer listserv who were less satisfied with the level of empathy, information provided, and quality of time spent with their oncologist were more likely to prefer the Internet as a primary source of health information (Tustin, 2010). In qualitative research, patients reported being motivated to seek health information online because they were disenchanted with the expertise, level of concern demonstrated, and quality of information received from their provider (Dolce, 2011). Beyond seeking information, patients with prostate cancer in another study reported that the outcomes of their Internet use were contingent on the receptivity of their health provider (Broom, 2005b). Those who felt encouraged by their provider to take an active role in decision making experienced greater empowerment from using the Internet for medical information. These findings stand in contrast to research in which no connection was found between patient-provider relations and patients' Internet use (Sciamanna, Clark, Diaz, & Newton, 2003).

Patient-provider relations are also connected with patients' Internet use in a second way. Patient information seeking may impact their relationship with providers. Patients in one study who felt reassured after acquiring health information online were more likely to report trusting their heath provider, being confident when interacting with him or her, and participating in joint decision making (Rider, Malik, & Chevassut, 2014). In another study, patients reported that seeking information allowed them to exercise power in their relationships with health care providers by becoming more knowledgeable and involved in decisions (Dolce, 2011). In focus groups with patients and providers, both groups indicated that information seeking online has led to changing roles and responsibilities (Townsend et al., 2015). Patients felt responsible for being knowledgeable about their health condition, and both groups felt that having informed patients could save time and allow for more interactive consultations. Yet challenges were also noted related to the burden of becoming informed and remaining open to more involved patients.

Beyond the quality of their interaction with providers, the effects of patients' Internet use appears to extend to the likelihood of even visiting a health provider. In one compelling test of this idea, C. Lee (2008) argued that health information available online displaces the need for similar information from providers. He predicted that Internet use would lead to reduced contact with health professionals for information but not influence physician visits for the purpose of treatment. In analyzing data from a two-wave survey of a nationally representative sample of U.S. citizens, his findings were unexpected. People who used the Internet for health information had increased contact with their health provider for medical information as well as treatment. As opposed to serving as a competing resource for information, Lee's (2008) results suggest that seeking information online may serve to make one's health more salient and reinforce the need for a health provider. Interviews with health information seekers underscore this possibility (Kivits, 2006). Patients reported that information acquired online was used to complement the information they received from medical professionals. In other research, patients who reported finding high-quality information online were more likely to agree with their providers and, in turn, comply with their provider's recommendations (Laugesen, Hassanein, & Yuan, 2015).

The timing of health information seeking by patients—whether before or after a medical consultation—offers insights about the connection between patient information seeking online and patient-provider relations. At least some patients appear to search for information online prior to visiting a health provider. In a survey of women at a gynecology outpatient clinic in England, approximately one-quarter of patients reported using the Internet for information related to their current issue prior to their visit (Neelapala, Duvvi, Kumar, & Kumar, 2008). The same percentage of patients with colorectal cancer reported using the Internet before visiting a health care provider about their symptoms (Thomson, Siminoff, & Longo, 2012). Although Internet users did not delay medical consultation relative to a comparison group, patients who searched for information online reported feeling somewhat more hesitant about discussing their symptoms with their health provider. In another study, information seeking before a visit left patients feeling better prepared to participate in the consultation and improved their interaction with providers (Kivits, 2006).

Several motivations and outcomes mark information seeking after a medical consultation. One group of researchers surveyed members of a large online health community and found that most respondents sought information online after their most recent provider visit (Bell, Hu, Orrange, & Kravitz, 2011; Li, Orrange, Kravitz, & Bell, 2014). Patients used a general search engine to look for information, read the contributions of support community members who had similar concerns, or visited an authoritative health website. The most common reason for seeking additional information was curiosity; less than one-third of the respondents did so because they received incomplete information from their provider or inadequate care. Several factors distinguished those patients who did and did not use the Internet to acquire additional information. Patients who were more worried after their visit, were less trusting of their physician, perceived the physician to be less patient-centered, generally used the Internet more frequently, and had greater levels of e-health literacy were all more likely to use the Internet for additional information after consultation.

Taken together, the preceding research offers fairly robust evidence to support the connection between patient-provider relations and patients' use of the Internet to acquire medical information. Patients who were less satisfied with their provider were more likely to seek information online, including after medical consultations. In the context of theory about patient-centered communication (Epstein et al., 2005; Stewart et al., 2000) and collaborative decision making (Politi & Street, 2011), these findings suggest that the Internet may be a viable alternative for patients who do not feel sufficiently understood or are otherwise unable to achieve shared understanding with their health care providers. Yet information seeking also allowed some patients to feel greater efficacy in their interactions with providers and more positively about their health providers. Patients who sought health information online in one longitudinal study were more likely to visit their provider in the future. Information seeking online appears to be a response and contributing factor to the quality of patient-provider relations.

Discussing Information from the Internet during Medical Consultations

One specific context in which patients' Internet use can have particularly important implications is during medical consultations. Patients may introduce information gleaned from the Internet during their visits with a health provider. Although this behavior has the potential to be beneficial, it can also present significant challenges for medical consultations and doctor-patient relations. In the following sections, the patient's perspective of this issue is first considered, followed by the perspective of health providers.

The Patient's Perspective

Although substantial variation exists in estimates regarding the volume of patients who discuss information acquired from the Internet with their health providers during medical consultations, such behavior appears to be fairly common. A survey conducted by the National Cancer Institute (2011) indicated that one-quarter of U.S. adults have talked with a health provider about medical information from the Internet. Commensurate findings have been reported in several other studies (Maloney et al., 2015; Schulz, Zufferey, & Hartung, 2011). For example, one-quarter of hematology patients (Rider et al., 2014), almost half of patients with breast cancer (D'Agostino et al., 2012), and half of patients surveyed from a family medicine practice (Liszka, Steyer, & Hueston, 2006) reported sharing or intending to share information acquired online during their consultation. In one study, questions about medical information from the Internet were the third most frequently addressed topic in patients' e-mails to health providers (Houston, Sands, Nash, & Ford, 2003). These findings may be contrasted with the results from research showing that other outside sources of health information are more prevalent than the Internet during medical consultations. Among a sample of cancer patients, information from family, friends, and other interpersonal sources was much more likely to be shared than information from the Internet (Lewis, Gray, Freres, & Hornik, 2009).

Patients have several motivations for discussing information acquired online with their health care provider. At the most general level, patients may believe that discussing Internet information allows them to get the most from their consultations (Bowes, Stevenson, Ahluwalia, & Murray, 2012). Four more specific motivations also have been identified and are summarized in table 6.2. The desire to learn more about their condition is one important motivation (D'Agostino et al., 2012; Sabee, Bylund, Weber, & Sonet, 2012). Sharing information acquired online during a consultation allows patients to become more knowledgeable about their condition and treatment. A second motivation for sharing Internet information with a health provider stems from the desire to seek advice and verification (D'Agostino et al., 2012; Sabee et al., 2012). Discussing Internet information makes it possible for patients to clarify specific concerns. Indeed, in one study, patients with breast cancer who intended to discuss information they found online with their provider experienced significantly higher levels of anxiety than individuals who did not intend to have such a discussion (D'Agostino et al., 2012). Demonstrating involvement is a third motivation (Bowes et al., 2012; D'Agostino et al., 2012; Sabee et al., 2012). Introducing

Table 6.2

Patients' Motivations for Sharing Internet Information with a Health Provider

Motivation	Description
Learning	Desire to become more knowledgeable about one's condition.
Advice/verification	Desire to receive feedback or clarification.
Demonstrating involvement	Desire to communicate one's investment and encourage the provider to take one seriously.
Provider evaluation	Desire to assess a provider's knowledge.

information from the Internet is an impression management tactic used to illustrate that patients are invested in their health and encourage the provider to take them and their concerns seriously. The desire to evaluate the knowledge of a health provider is a final motivation for introducing Internet information during a consultation (Sabee et al., 2012). Patients may share information as a means to assess the scope of their provider's medical knowledge.

There are also several reasons that patients may refrain from sharing information acquired online during a medical consultation. One major concern listed by patients involves challenging their health provider's authority (Bowes et al., 2012; Chiu, 2011; Silver, 2015; Sommerhalder, Abraham, Zufferey, Barth, & Abel, 2009). Patients are concerned that sharing information could be seen as an affront to their provider. Patients also withhold information when it is consistent with their provider's evaluation (Sommerhalder et al., 2009). Other reasons for not sharing include trusting one's provider and because the information was only acquired for the purpose of personal learning (D'Agostino et al., 2012) as well as a lack of time during the consultation (Kirschning & von Kardorff, 2008). Older adults may withhold information acquired online to avoid embarrassment stemming from difficulties understanding or explaining the information (Silver, 2015).

The range of strategies used by patients to introduce Internet information during medical consultations is fairly limited. Almost half of the respondents in one study presented the information to their health provider in the form of direct questions (Bylund, Gueguen, D'Agostino, Li, & Sonet, 2010). Making suggestions based on the information and bringing in printed copies of webpages were two additional strategies reported in other studies (Kirschning & von Kardorff, 2008; Sommerhalder et al., 2009). Once the topic has been raised, patients tend to discuss information directly related to their condition and care with providers. Among patients with cancer, information about prognosis was common along with information related to treatments, alternative therapies, diagnosis, and clinical trials (Bylund et al., 2010; Maloney et al., 2015). Almost half of the respondents discussed information from formal cancer organization websites such as the site hosted by the American Cancer Society. WebMD.com was another common source, along with websites operated by hospitals, governmental agencies, and foundations.

Patients who introduced Internet information during a medical consultation reported a variety of responses from their providers. Positive responses included providers being open to the information and providing feedback, whereas negative responses involved having the information dismissed or the doctor communicating an unwillingness to consider it (Bowes et al., 2012). A survey conducted by the National Cancer Institute (2011) showed that more than two-thirds of respondents who discussed medical information from the Internet reported feeling that their doctor was somewhat or very interested. Yet one-quarter of the respondents felt that their doctor was only a little or not at all interested. Other researchers have reported similar findings (Kirschning & von Kardorff, 2008; Newnham et al., 2006). Although more than three-quarters of respondents in one study felt that their doctor took the information seriously, almost one-fifth noted that their doctor disagreed with them or the information (Bylund et al., 2010). Less than 5 percent indicated that their doctor was dismissive of the information or issued a warning about acquiring information online. Other researchers have examined the attributions made by patients about their provider's response to Internet information shared during a consultation. A group of patients with cancer and their caregivers attributed their providers' responses to their knowledge of the field (or lack thereof), (in)flexibility in their approach to treatments or interpretations, and (un)willingness to collaborate (Sabee et al., 2012).

Provider responses to Internet information shared by patients during medical consultations can have consequences for doctor-patient relations. At least 40 percent of patients at a hematology clinic indicated that sharing Internet information with their provider improved their confidence, led them to ask more questions, and improved their ability to make joint decisions (Rider et al., 2014). Similar findings were reported in a study of patients with cancer (Bylund et al., 2010). Patients were less likely to want to change providers when their provider acted interested or took the information seriously. Taking the information seriously also made patients feel more satisfied, whereas disagreements made them feel less satisfied. Yet other researchers found no differences in those patients who did and did not discuss online medical information with their provider in terms of satisfaction with the visit, trust in the physician, or change in anxiety (D'Agostino et al., 2012). Similarly, more than half of patients recruited from the hematology clinic reported that sharing Internet information had little impact on their consultation (Rider et al., 2014).

The Provider's Perspective

Although much of the scholarship examining the introduction of Internet information during a medical consultation tends to focus on patients, researchers have begun to study this issue from the health providers' perspective. One primary objective has been to better understand how health providers perceive and respond to Internet-informed patients. A great deal of variation exists in provider perceptions, ranging from those who recognize the promise of informed patients to others who are extremely wary.

Across several studies, researchers have consistently reported that at least some health providers view patients' health-related Internet use negatively (Ahluwalia, Murray, Stevenson, Kerr, & Burns, 2010; Broom, 2005a; Caiata-Zufferey & Schulz, 2012). One group of scholars interviewed general practitioners and found that patients' use of the Internet to acquire health information was generally seen as a "potential nuisance" that made their role more complex (Caiata-Zufferey & Schulz, 2012, p. 741). In another study, informed patients were described as a threat to the medical authority of some specialists (Broom, 2005a). These physicians preferred more passive patients and appealed to the dangers of Internet information as a disciplining strategy. During consultations, the introduction of Internet information by patients was a source of anxiety for the general practitioners interviewed in one study (Ahluwalia et al., 2010). These physicians were concerned about their potential to lose control of the interaction along with being undervalued or perceived as incompetent. They also described attempting to overcome these feelings and demonstrate that they were open to the information acquired by patients. Some doctors even explicitly admitted a lack of knowledge to patients.

Other health providers, in contrast, welcomed Internet-informed patients (Broom, 2005a; Sommerhalder et al., 2009). Some physicians believed that having knowledgeable patients made it possible to discuss medical issues in greater detail (Sommerhalder et al., 2009). Specialists felt that health-related Internet use by patients could improve medical care by allowing patients to take greater responsibility for and become more involved in their care (Broom, 2005a). These specialists believed that informed patients were more likely to feel positively about and comply with treatment instructions.

When medical information is introduced by patients during consultations, health providers may respond in one of several different ways. Caiata-Zufferey and Schulz (2012) interviewed physicians and reported four primary strategies. Resisting involved attempts to ignore or devalue the information. Physicians who pursued this strategy tended to view health information as a potential danger to patients and something that undermines the job of a medical professional. Repairing strategies consisted of evaluating the information and warning patients about its limitations. Providers using this strategy considered health information as something that should be delivered solely by medical professionals. Co-construction strategies involved using the information as a springboard for discussion. Health providers who used this strategy saw the potential value in health information as long as it was eventually discussed with a medical professional. Their goal was to create a consensus about diagnoses and treatments. Finally, enhancement strategies involved doctors encouraging patients to be proactive and giving them tools to acquire high-quality information. Health providers who enacted this strategy tended to view any source that provides high-quality information as valuable and felt that patients ultimately were responsible for their health care decisions.

In some instances, providers may even actively encourage patients to acquire health information online. In one survey of cancer patients, almost half reported receiving referrals from their providers to other sources of information, although patients were referred specifically to the Internet infrequently (Lewis et al., 2009). In a study of general practitioners in Australia, more than half recommended health websites to their patients (Usher, 2011). The most common reasons for doing so were to help educate patients and enhance their relationship with patients. Most of the recommendations involved webpages dedicated to specific diseases. Another group of researchers conducted a novel experiment to examine the effects of Internet referrals by doctors. Patients recently diagnosed with carpal tunnel syndrome were randomly assigned to receive a handout directing them to a foundation webpage focused on the health condition or to a control group that received no such recommendation (Aung, Wu, Tokumi, Kuo, & Day, 2015). Almost half of the respondents who received the handout visited the webpage. However, there were no differences in knowledge of carpal tunnel or satisfaction with their health provider between the groups that did and did not receive the handout or between participants who did and did not access the foundation website. The Internet referral had little impact on patients.

In summary, a fair amount has been learned about the introduction of Internet information by patients during medical consultations. Studies of patients suggest that this behavior is relatively common, and gaining information about one's condition is a primary motivation. This is important because it signals a sense of agency and desire for involvement among patients, which has been linked with beneficial health outcomes (Street, Makoul, Arora, & Epstein, 2009). Patients also introduced medical information as a means to demonstrate their commitment and to test their provider's knowledge. Patient reports indicate that doctors tend to respond positively, and tentative evidence links positive responses with patient satisfaction. Yet research on providers reflects a tension in the way that these two groups view the Internet. Providers' perceptions of Internet-informed patients and the introduction of Internet information during consultations were mixed. Some providers welcomed more knowledgeable patients, whereas others viewed them as a threat to their authority. These findings suggest that, for at least some health providers, online health information and informed patients may represent a challenge to traditional roles (Broom, 2005b; Hardey, 2001). More broadly, such findings underscore some challenges to achieving the ideals of patient-centeredness (Epstein et al., 2005; Stewart et al., 2000) and shared decision making (Charles et al., 1997; Politi & Street, 2011).

Patient-Provider E-mail

Beyond the context of medical consultations, the use and effects of e-mail between patients and providers has been a longstanding topic of interest. In giving patients and providers additional opportunities to communicate, e-mail is proposed to allow providers to better understand their patients and patients to better manage their health condition(s). Existing research does not offer much evidence to suggest that the promise of e-mail has been realized.

Ye, Rust, Fry-Johnson, and Strothers (2010) conducted a systematic review of 24 studies and reported a consistent trend regarding patient-provider e-mail. Although many patients expressed interest in e-mailing their health care provider, the opportunity to do so has been relatively rare. In a survey of WebMD.com users conducted around the year 2000, for example, only 6 percent of active e-mail users communicated with their health provider using this technology, but almost two-thirds indicated the desire for such interaction (Sittig, King, & Hazlehurst, 2001). A survey of older adults conducted during 2003 showed that only 1 percent of respondents had communicated with a health provider vie e-mail, but more than half were enthusiastic about the prospect. Almost half of the sample in another study even indicated a willingness to pay for e-mail access to their health providers (Virji et al., 2006). These trends appear to hold in research conducted more recently. In a survey of pediatric caregivers, more than three-quarters of respondents reported that they would like to communicate with their doctor via e-mail, but only 10 percent indicated having done so (Dudas & Crocetti, 2013). An exception can be found in the results of a survey conducted by the National Cancer Institute (2013). Almost 30 percent of respondents who used the Internet reported using e-mail to communicate with a doctor or doctor's office during 2013. Further, researchers examining the National Cancer Institute's data showed that e-mail interaction between patients and health providers has increased since 2003 (Prestin, Vieux, & Chou, 2015).

Although many people desire to communicate with their health care provider via e-mail, sizeable groups also feel differently. Only about half of the respondents in a national survey were willing to communicate health goals and test results with their doctor via e-mail, whereas three-quarters or more were willing to do so using the telephone (Jenssen, Mitra, Shah, Wan, & Grande, 2016). In a study examining low-income patients from primary care clinics in Texas, most respondents did not want to use e-mail, text messaging, or the Internet to send and receive information from their health provider (Hill, Burge, Haring, & Young, 2012). Other researchers have found that many patients who have the opportunity do not actually e-mail their health provider. Patients referred to a single surgeon during a one-year period were given access to e-mail and told that e-mail was the surgeon's preferred communication mode (Ketteridge, Delbridge, & Delbridge, 2005). Only 16 percent of patients e-mailed the surgeon. At a pediatric rheumatology practice, 40 percent of the more than 300 families that were given access e-mailed the physician over a two-year period (P. Rosen & Kwoh, 2007).

Despite the small proportion of patients who have communicated with a health provider via e-mail, it appears that doctors do e-mail (some of) their patients. Estimates of physician e-mail use, however, vary widely. In a survey of physicians at an outpatient clinic conducted around the year 2000, almost three-quarters of the physicians indicated using e-mail to communicate with patients (Gaster et al., 2003). In surveys conducted during 2005 and 2008, 17 percent and 20 percent of physicians indicated sending e-mails to patients from their practices (Menachemi, Prickett, & Brooks, 2011). Half of the physicians in a survey conducted during 2009 indicated using e-mail to communicate with patients (Cooper et al., 2012). It may be that doctors are selective about the patients with whom they are willing to exchange e-mail. A survey of physicians showed that, although two-thirds reported using e-mail to communicate with patients, they only did so with less than 5 percent of patients (Pizziferri et al., 2003). A key issue for physicians in another study was selecting the patients to be given e-mail access (Patt, Houston, Jenckes, Sands, & Ford, 2003). Yet the physicians interviewed did not appear to have any clear strategies for making selections, beyond that patients have Internet access.

When they offer e-mail access to patients, the volume of e-mail received by providers from patients appears to be fairly modest. Several researchers have found that doctors received approximately one to three messages from patients per day. One pediatric rheumatologist, for example, received an average of 1.2 e-mail messages per day over a two-year period (Rosen & Kwoh, 2007). During that time period, the average amount of time the doctor spent per e-mail (132.1 seconds) was less than the amount of time spent on the average phone call (309.2 seconds). In other research, patients at a pain clinic produced approximately 3 messages per day over an eight-month period (Ruiz, García, & Riquelme, 2014), and five physicians each received a little more than one message per day over the course of one month (Sittig, 2003). The preceding results can be contrasted with another study in which a sample of physicians reported receiving a single e-mail message every four days (Gaster et al., 2003)

Use of e-mail for patient-provider communication varies depending on several factors. Among patients, education appears to be important. Patients who were more educated were more likely to have e-mail access to a health provider (Beckjord et al., 2007; Lee et al., 2016; Prestin et al., 2015; Santana et al., 2010). Beyond education, patients who were younger or had a chronic condition (Lee et al., 2016), were in poorer health (Prestin et al., 2015), had a regular health provider (Beckjord et al., 2007), or lived in an urban area (Beckjord et al., 2007; Prestin et al., 2015) were more likely to e-mail a health provider. Among health providers, working in a larger practice (Brooks & Menachemi, 2006) as well as being female, a specialist, or having a greater level of computer competence (Menachemi et al., 2011) were predictors of e-mail use with patients. Beyond demographics, the quality of patients' existing relationship with their provider proved critical in one qualitative study (Andreassen, Trondsen, Kummervold, Gammon, & Hjortdahl, 2006). Having a high level of trust in a health provider helped to ensure that e-mail was successful from the patients' perspectives.

Both patients and providers report several benefits of e-mail. Patients in two studies indicated that e-mail made it easier to contact their health provider and discuss things that were omitted during consultations due to time constraints (Andreassen et al., 2006; Leong, Gingrich, Lewis, Mauger, & George, 2005). Most caregivers in another study reported feeling that e-mail increased their access to the provider, improved the quality of communication with the provider, and helped to reduce their fears and concerns (Rosen & Kwoh, 2007). Providers reported similar benefits in several studies. Interviews with physicians indicated that e-mail made them more accessible to patients (Patt et al., 2003). E-mail has been deemed helpful in reducing the volume of care by making it easier—particularly relative to the telephone—to address routine or noncritical issues (Gaster et al., 2003; Houston et al., 2003; Patt et al., 2003). E-mail was even seen by physicians as having the potential to improve their relationship with patients (Moyer, Stern, Dobias, Cox, & Katz, 2002).

In addition to the benefits, several limitations of e-mail have been identified. More than one-third of patients in one study reported that they would rather speak to a "real person" or call their doctor on the telephone than use e-mail (Moyer et al., 2002). Providers were concerned with the potential burden of patient e-mails and, in particular, the time demands (Houston et al., 2003; Patt et al., 2003). Other limitations included patients' ability to use e-mail appropriately (Houston et al., 2003) and concerns with security (Moyer et al., 2002).

The American Medical Association (AMA) and the American Medical Informatics Association (AMIA) have developed guidelines for patient-provider e-mail. They include informing patients about privacy issues, establishing a turn-around time for messages, along with several other recommendations. In two studies, most physicians rarely conformed to many of these guidelines. Less than 10 percent in the study adhered to at least half of the 14 guidelines developed by the AMA and AMIA (Brooks & Menachemi, 2006). In a survey targeting a similar population three years later, adherence remained low (Menachemi et al., 2011). The most frequently followed guideline involved including printed copies of patients' e-mail messages in their records; this guideline was adhered to by approximately one-third of the sample.

The content of patient-provider e-mail focuses on a relatively limited range of issues. Ye and colleagues' (2010) systematic review offers several insights. E-mail messages tend to address informational content related to treatment and medication (Andersen & Ruland, 2009; Leong et al., 2005; Ruiz et al., 2014; Sittig, 2003; White, Moyer, Stern, & Katz, 2004). In a study of e-mails sent from providers to patients in a diabetes intervention, for example, almost half included information and advice or requested information from patients (Robinson, Turner, Levine, & Tian, 2011). The informational nature of e-mail is further evidenced by the fact that fewer than half of all messages received by physicians in one study were determined to require a follow-up, such as with a prescription renewal (White et al., 2004). These uses of e-mail by patients and providers generally align with reports of what physicians view as appropriate. Half or more of the physicians in one study indicated that e-mail was appropriate for scheduling an appointment, refilling medication, relaying normal tests result, and answering questions about disease management (Gaster et al., 2003).

Researchers have also examined the content of e-mail messages exchanged by patients and health providers at more microscopic levels. Messages from physicians tend to be relatively short. Across two studies, physician replies ranged from an average of 39 words (Sittig, 2003) to 62 words (Roter, Larson, Sands, Ford, & Houston, 2008). Messages were returned to patients fairly quickly. Most physicians in two studies replied within one day of receiving a patient's e-mail message (Leong et al., 2005; Sittig, 2003). Perhaps not surprisingly, e-mail messages did not typically address urgent issues (Anand, Feldman, Geller, Bisbee, & Bauchner, 2005; White et al., 2004). Only 6 percent of all messages examined in one study addressed urgent matters such as a disease flare or new symptoms (Rosen & Kwoh, 2007).

Although relatively little research has been conducted to examine the outcomes of patient-provider e-mail, tentative evidence suggests that such interactions may have concrete benefits for patients' health. In one experimental study, a group of physicians was randomly assigned to offer e-mail access to patients or serve as a control group without e-mail (Leong et al., 2005). Relative to the control group, patients who could e-mail their provider reported a significantly greater increase in their satisfaction with the convenience and amount of time spent with their physician. Commensurate findings were reported by researchers surveying physicians who frequently used e-mail to communicate with their patients (Houston et al., 2003). Most providers reported being satisfied with e-mail.

Beyond satisfaction, patient-provider e-mail has been linked with beneficial changes in patients' health and health behavior. In one study, the number of messages sent from providers to patients in a diabetes intervention was associated with patients' frequency of glucose monitoring (Robinson et al., 2011). Patients with diabetes in the intervention who received a greater number of e-mail messages monitored their blood glucose more frequently. Another group of scholars examined the implications of e-mail access on the physiological functioning of patients with diabetes and hypertension (Zhou, Kanter, Wang, & Garrido, 2010). Compared with a matched control group that did not use e-mail, patients with diabetes who e-mailed their doctor during the previous two months experienced significantly greater improvements in glycemic control, cholesterol, and blood pressure. Notably, the researchers also found some evidence consistent with a dose-response effect. Patients who e-mailed their doctor about two separate events tended to fare better than those who only e-mailed their doctor once.

Taken as a whole, several conclusions can be drawn from research examining e-mail use among patients and health providers. Demand for e-mail access to health providers outstrips supply. Whereas relatively few patients have the ability to e-mail their health care provider, sizeable numbers desire the opportunity for such access. A noteworthy number of providers use e-mail for communicating with patients, but they appear to be doing so selectively. The potential for e-mail to make providers more accessible was recognized as a key benefit by both providers and patients. Providers, however, are concerned with the potential burden created by e-mail. Most e-mail messages tend to focus on what might be considered informational topics related to treatment and care, with urgent issues being rare. The outcomes of patient-provider e-mail are largely unknown. Although some initial evidence suggests that e-mail may improve patients' satisfaction and health behavior, little research has been conducted to address this issue.

Health Providers and Communication Technologies

Although e-mail has received most of the attention from researchers studying patient-provider interaction, the implications of several other communication technologies for health providers have been considered. Providers' use of social media has been one topic of interest. Providers appear to be making limited use of social media for professional purposes. A second topic involves physician evaluation websites, which are fairly widely used by patients. Scholarship on each of these topics will be reviewed in the following sections.

Providers' Social Media Use

Use of social media as a professional resource among health providers is fairly limited. Although evidence indicates that some physicians use social media in their personal lives, professional uses of these technologies do not appear to be widespread (Bosslet, Torke, Hickman, Terry, & Helft, 2011). Less than one-third of the residents, junior physicians, and senior physicians in one study reported having a professional social media account, and one-fifth or fewer reported using social media to acquire medical news (Klee, Covey, & Zhong, 2015). Among a sample of Canadian urologists, fewer than 10 percent reported using social media daily or frequently for professional reasons (Fuoco & Leveridge, 2015). These findings are consistent with a survey of community pharmacists in which less than 10 percent reported communicating with other health care professionals or patients using the SNS Facebook or microblog Twitter (Shcherbakova & Shepherd, 2014). The preceding results stand in contrast to the findings from a survey of primary care physicians and oncologists, in which more than half reported using social media weekly or more frequently for acquiring medical information and almost half reported contributing to social media as frequently (McGowan et al., 2012).

Providers do not appear to be overly optimistic about the potential of social media in medical care. Only one-fifth of practicing physicians in one study felt that SNSs had the potential to improve provider-patient communication (Bosslet et al., 2011). However, some uses of social media have been consistently deemed more and less acceptable by health providers. The most widely accepted use of social media in one study was as a means to present information about one's medical practice (Fuoco & Leveridge, 2015). Among a sample of physicians in the Netherlands, for example, Twitter and LinkedIn were most frequently used for marketing and communicating with colleagues (Antheunis, Tates, & Nieboer, 2013). Connecting with patients has been generally viewed as inappropriate. Less than 10 percent (Klee et al., 2015) or 5 percent (Brown, Ryan, & Harris, 2014) of the health providers surveyed in two studies were willing to accept a "friend request" from a patient on an SNS. Despite their disapproval, some health providers report being contacted by patients. One-third of providers in one study who used an SNS (Bosslet et al., 2011) and one-fifth of providers in another study (Brown et al., 2014) had received a "friend request" from a patient or a patient's family member.

Providers also registered other concerns about social media use. Use of social media to surveil patients was one specific disapproved of activity. Across two studies, one-fifth or fewer of the providers reported that it was acceptable to review publicly available information about patients online as part of normal patient care (Bosslet et al., 2011; Brown et al., 2014). Even in the case of an emergency such as a suicide attempt, only one-third of providers felt that it would be appropriate to review a patient's social media account (Brown et al., 2014). More broadly, most health providers in another study reported that unprofessional activity on social media could lead to professional disciplinary action or recognized the need for regulatory bodies to adapt to this new environment (Fuoco & Leveridge, 2015). Yet professional training related to social media use does not appear to be widespread. Less than one-third of providers in one study had received any formal training in professional social media use, and less than half reported that their hospital had a social media policy (Klee et al., 2015).

Tentative evidence suggests that physicians' social media use could impact their relationships with patients. One group of researchers randomly assigned members of the public and medical students to view and evaluate the profile of an SNS user identified as a medical student (Jain et al., 2014). The profiles were manipulated to include images depicting several different activities, and participants were asked to report their comfort with having the profile owner serve as their doctor in the future. Relative to medical students, members of the public were significantly less comfortable having a future doctor who had posted images of marijuana use, alcohol use, partying, or romantic relationships. The results from this study underscore the potential for social media use to influence patients' perceptions and the patient-provider relationship.

Provider Evaluation Websites

Provider evaluation websites are clearinghouses where individual patients can publicly rate their health providers. Patients typically are asked to answer a series of closed-ended items and then include any comments they have about their provider. This information is then aggregated and made available to website visitors.

More than 40 percent of U.S. adults are estimated to have consulted online evaluations for health providers, medical facilities, or a particular drug or treatment (Thackeray, Crookston, & West, 2013). Almost 10 percent have contributed such a review. People who consulted an online medical review were more likely to have a chronic disease, see a regular health provider, have more education, earn a greater income, live in an urban area, and be female. Beyond self-report data from patients, more objective evidence exists to illustrate the popularity of physician evaluation websites. As of 2010, almost one-fifth of practicing U.S. physicians had appeared on a provider evaluation website (Gao, McCullough, Agarwal, & Jha, 2012). In a random sample of 250 physicians identified from a national directory of hand surgeons, all but 5 had at least one rating on one of the three popular provider evaluation websites (Trehan, DeFrancesco, Nguyen, Charalel, & Daluiski, 2016).

Physician ratings on evaluation websites tend to be fairly positive. One group of researchers evaluated the 10 most visited evaluation websites and analyzed almost 5,000 ratings (Kadry, Chu, Kadry, Gammas, & Macario, 2011). The median rating on websites using a 100-point evaluation scale (with higher scores indicating a more positive rating) was 76. Moreover, more than 60 percent of reviews had a rating of 75 or higher. On websites that used a 5-point scale, the median rating was 4, and almost 60 percent of reviews had a rating of 4 or higher. In another study, mean ratings for a random sample of hand surgeons were consistently high across three provider evaluation websites (Trehan et al., 2016). The lowest mean score for all physicians on one of the three websites was 3.8 out of 5 stars.

A broad range of topics are addressed in patient reviews. Six themes were identified in an analysis of reviews submitted by patients who had seen their doctor for at least one year (Detz, López, & Sarkar, 2013). The most common topic involved the personality of the physician, including his or her empathy and overall excellence. The remaining topics included the physician's technical competence, communication skills, accessibility, staff/office environment, and coordination of care. Other researchers have found that the valence of patient comments varied based on the specific topic being evaluated. Whereas positive comments tended to focus on provider-dependent factors such as competence and communication, negative comments were more likely to address topics such as the office staff or cost (Trehan et al., 2016). An analysis of nine online review sites focusing on surgeons who performed one of three types of procedures showed differences in the content of ratings based on the relative activity level of the surgeons (Segal et al., 2012). Relative to surgeons who performed fewer procedures, those who performed more procedures received more reviews and comments, had a greater proportion of positive reviews about the quality of their care, and had a smaller proportion of negative reviews about quality of care.

Relatively limited research has been conducted to determine whether and how physician evaluation websites influence patients' perceptions and behavior. One group of scholars examined the effects of different types of information included in provider evaluations (Kanouse, Schlesinger, Shaller, Martino, & Rybowski, 2016). Some participants only saw numeric evaluations of providers, whereas others also had access to patient comments. Although there were no differences in patients' perceptions of the website or their satisfaction with the providers available, notable discrepancies occurred in website use and the nature of the provider that patients selected. When comments were present, patients spent more time reviewing the website but were more likely to select a lower-performing clinician. This effect was stronger when a larger number of doctors were available to be evaluated.

In other experimental research, scholars examined the effects of the proportion and order of negative and positive reviews on evaluations of providers (Li, Feng, Chen, & Bell, 2015). They found that participants' willingness to be treated by the physician decreased as the proportion of negative comments increased. They also reported tentative evidence that participants were less willing to be treated when negative comments appeared prior to positive comments than vice versa. The results from these two experimental studies underscore the potential effects of physician evaluation websites on patients.

Several conclusions can be gleaned from research examining physicians' use of social media and provider evaluation websites. Use of social media for professional purposes by health providers has not been widespread. Moreover, providers tend to be pessimistic about its prospects in medical care. Provider evaluation websites, however, are fairly widely used by patients. Provider reviews tend to be positive and focus on factors such as the provider's personality, technical competence, communication skills, and office environment. Tentative evidence suggests that such reviews can impact patients' perceptions of providers.

Issues Warranting Greater Attention in Patient-Provider Research

Although existing research has revealed several important insights, much remains to be learned about the uses and effects of communication technologies among patients and health care providers. All of the issues addressed in this chapter would benefit from additional study. Yet several specific topics might be privileged. First, additional research would be valuable to explore the connection between the quality of patients' relationships with their health care provider and use of the Internet for information seeking. Patient information seeking appears to be a product of and contribute to their relationship with their health provider. Integrating theory about cooperative decision making (Politi & Street, 2011) could yield important insights. It would also be worthwhile to further investigate Internet use before and after a medical consultation. The types of sources visited by health information seekers are particularly important to consider. Visiting an online support community or blog to learn about others' experiences may result in different expectations and responses to providers than does searching for medical information on health websites.

A second issue meriting greater attention involves the role and consequences of introducing Internet information during a medical consultation. Building from existing research on patients' motivations for sharing online information, it would be valuable to further examine the mechanics and effects of such sharing. The ways in which Internet information is introduced in terms of the timing, presentation, and justifications are important to consider. Sabee and colleagues' (2012) work examining patients' interaction goals provides a valuable theoretical starting point for such an endeavor. It would also be beneficial to further explore the outcomes of introducing online information. Important questions remain about how this behavior impacts patient-provider relations and the quality of medical consultations.

Additional research would be valuable to better understand the outcomes of patient-provider e-mail. Researchers have documented trends in e-mail use, the types of content shared, and general responses of patients and providers. Although such information is certainly valuable, it is also important to examine the outcomes of e-mail use. It largely remains to be seen whether e-mail use between patients and providers improves relationship quality or patients' ability to cope with illness. Moreover, the theoretical mechanisms that might bring about such effects deserve greater consideration. It seems possible that e-mail may be beneficial to patients by providing additional information that directly allows them to manage their health condition more effectively as well as indirectly by increasing their trust and satisfaction with their provider. Addressing these issues is critical to fully understanding, and possibly realizing, the potential of e-mail in this context.

A final issue warranting additional attention in scholarship examining the implications of communication technologies for patients and providers involves providers' use of social media. Contemporary research suggests that providers' use of social media for professional purposes is not widespread, and providers generally fail to see its utility in this context. Given this state of affairs, it would be valuable to explore the conditions under which—if any—providers' social media use could improve patient-provider relations or health delivery. Social media may have an unforeseen potential to benefit patients and health providers.

Conclusion

Researchers studying the implications of communication technologies for patient-provider interactions and relationships have uncovered several noteworthy trends. Patients' health-related communication technology use appears to be connected to the quality of their relationship with their heath provider. Patients who are less satisfied are more likely to seek out health information online. During medical consultations, patients introduce medical information from the Internet in an effort to learn more about their condition but also to demonstrate their involvement and evaluate their provider's knowledge. A great deal of variation exists in provider responses to Internet-informed patients. Patients who desire e-mail access to their provider vastly outnumber patients who have such an opportunity. Use of social media for professional purposes by providers is not widespread, and providers are pessimistic about its potential to improve patient care. Although these conclusions highlight the importance of communication technologies in patient-provider relationships, they are based on a relatively limited number of studies and should be considered as tentative. Future research is essential to more fully explore these issues and, as a result, refine our understanding of the implications of patient-provider communication for digital coping.

7 End of Life and Bereavement

Facing the end of life can be traumatic. Although everyone will eventually die, serious illness can serve to heighten the salience of one's morality. Patients may experience existential anxieties about the meaning of life and their legacy. The quality of patients' remaining days or months may be a significant concern as might the long-term well-being of family and friends. Death also creates significant challenges for the bereaved. In addition to coping with the loss of a loved one, the bereaved may be tasked with carrying out the deceased's final wishes.

The thesis of this chapter is that communication technologies have important implications for the end of life and bereavement. The chapter begins with background information about end-of-life and bereavement communication. The use of communication technologies at the end of life is next considered, followed by a discussion of digital bereavement and mourning. The chapter concludes with a review of issues warranting attention in research on communication technologies at the end of life and in bereavement.

End of Life and Bereavement

Fundamentals of End-of-Life and Bereavement Communication
Prior to discussing the implications of communication technologies, it is first important to discuss some basic properties of end-of-life and bereavement communication. Although the end of life has been defined in different ways, the definition adopted in this chapter involves any point between when a person is diagnosed with a terminal illness and his or her death (Keeley, 2015). From the patient's perspective, end-of-life care can be distinguished by five dimensions (Singer, Martin, & Kelner, 1999). Two

dimensions address physical issues associated with dying, including adequate symptom management and avoiding any undesired prolongation of life. Yet the remaining three dimensions are social in nature. The end of life can involve the desire to gain control over decisions made about one's care, dispense burden that dying and death may impose on one's friends and family members, and strengthen relationships with loved ones.

Death is typically marked by a series of social rituals. Funerals offer an important means to commemorate the deceased's life and begin providing closure for the bereaved (Kunkel & Dennis, 2003). Eulogies are one important way of memorializing the dead. Eulogies involve a public speech commemorating the life of the deceased that can serve several sophisticated functions. Jamieson and Campbell (1982) explain that, as a rhetorical form, eulogies "acknowledge the death, transform the relationship between the living and the deceased from present to past tense, ease the mourner's terror at confronting their own mortality, console them by arguing that the deceased lives on, and reknit the community" (p. 147). In other words, eulogies generally serve to recognize the deceased, console survivors, and preserve the broader communities in which the deceased was a member.

Bereavement refers to the general state of having experienced the loss of someone close. The bereaved can face a number of challenges (Cowles & Rodgers, 1991). Several models have been developed to explain the bereavement process (for a review, see Stroebe & Schut, 2001). In the dual-process model of coping with bereavement (Stroebe & Schut, 1999, 2010), two general classes of stressors are identified. Loss-oriented stressors involve the loss experience such as feelings of grief. Restoration-oriented stressors are secondary stressors that pertain to remaking one's life without the deceased. Acclimating to new roles and responsibilities such as managing the family checkbook are examples of restoration-oriented stressors. Bereavement is conceptualized as an ongoing process involving oscillation between confronting and avoiding loss and restoration-oriented stressors.

Affordances of Communication Technologies at the End of Life
Various communication technologies have historically played a role in death and dying. Cave paintings and drawings were used by early humans to memorialize the dead (S. Jones, 2004). Written memorials on gravestones and newspaper obituary sections are more recent technological means used

to remember the deceased (P. Roberts & Vidal, 2000). By the mid-1990s, videophones were being used by health providers to deliver end-of-life care to terminally ill patients in their own homes (Doolittle, Yaezel, Otto, & Clemens, 1998). In recent years, memorials for the deceased have appeared on social network sites (SNSs) (P. Roberts, 2012). Four affordances of communication technologies are particularly relevant at the end of life and in bereavement: reach, notification, documentation, and visibility. Each of these four factors is summarized in table 7.1.

The affordance of reach involves the potential to use communication technologies to share the same message with a group of people simultaneously. This affordance is critical at the end of life and during bereavement because it allows family members to disseminate information efficiently in terms of time and emotional resources. Discussing end-of-life issues can be difficult, and the obligation to share the same information repeatedly to update an entire social network can be incredibly taxing emotionally (Ferguson, Massimi, Crist, & Moffatt, 2014). Using e-mail, SNSs, or other technologies, it is possible for patients or their loved ones to reach a potentially vast audience with a single communication attempt. This affordance can also be valuable among the bereaved in activities such as coordinating funeral arrangements (Moncur, Bikker, Kasket, & Troyer, 2012).

Notification is a second affordance of communication technologies for end-of-life communication. This affordance involves the potential to leave a message for a person or group in which a response is not required or expected. Communication technologies that allow notification are important because they allow survivors to construct messages directed at the deceased. Online memorial websites and SNS memorials are used by mourners to convey messages to the dead (Walter, Hourizi, Moncur, &

Table 7.1
Key Affordances of Communication Technologies at the End of Life

Affordance	Definition
Reach	Potential to connect and communicate with a specific group of people simultaneously.
Notification	Potential to leave a message for someone in which a response is neither required nor expected.
Documentation	Potential to create a lasting record of one's thoughts, feelings, and experiences.
Visibility	Potential to witness the behaviors of others.

Pitsillides, 2011). Although it seems likely that most users are aware that the dead cannot directly respond to their messages, the notification affordance offers a way for mourners to continue their connection with the deceased.

Documentation is a third affordance that involves the potential to leave a lasting record of one's discourse. One's legacy may be a salient concern at the end of life (Chiu & Hsieh, 2013). The potential to display one's messages permanently offered by some communication technologies such as blogs makes it possible to document one's thoughts, beliefs, and experiences for survivors. It is possible to create a written record that could be accessed and read by one's friends and family after one's death. Such a record could help survivors cope with their loss and be a means of constructing one's legacy.

Visibility is a final affordance of communication technologies that is important at the end of life and in bereavement. Visibility refers to the potential to be observed or witness the behaviors of others. Grieving in online memorial websites, SNS memorials, and online grief support communities is a public behavior. One's contributions are available to other visitors, and one may see the messages left by others. The visibility of mourning and bereavement is important because it underscores the social nature of these activities (Jackson & Usher, 2015; Walter et al., 2011). Like at a funeral or wake, the norms for mourning are socially (re)constructed in these contexts and may have a communal component.

Communication Technologies at the End of Life

With background information about end-of-life communication in place, it is possible to examine the implications of communication technologies in this context. Three areas where communication technologies play an important role include hospice and telehospice care, communicating about the end of life, and in patients' digital remains after their death. Each of these topics will be addressed in the following sections.

Hospice Care and Telehospice

Communication technologies can play an important role in hospice or palliative care, which involves patients who are seriously or terminally ill. In case studies of patients receiving palliative care and their families, the Internet was an important resource for acquiring health information (Pereira, Bruera, Macmillan, & Kavanagh, 2000). In some instances, Internet use made it possible to identify beneficial treatment strategies. In other cases, information acquired online conflicted with health care provider recommendations or led patients to request alternate treatments or treatment centers. Other researchers interviewing the friends and family members of recently deceased patients in hospice found that, although face-to-face interaction tended to be favored, communication technologies were beneficial in a number of instances (Ferguson et al., 2014). Wireless devices were valuable to extend the independence of patients in hospice, and text messaging was seen as valuable among family members to maintain emotional distance from their loved one. E-mail and SNSs were used with mixed success by family members to coordinate people and transmit routine information.

The implications of communication technologies extend beyond patients to hospice caregivers and health professionals. A survey of palliative care professionals showed that most respondents used the Internet to acquire clinical information or access online medical journals, and more than half subscribed to a listserv or newsgroup dedicated to palliative care (Pereira, Bruera, & Quan, 2001). Almost 15 percent reported consulting with other professionals online, and 6 percent counseled patients online. More recently, researchers conducting a systematic review identified several distinct users of communication technologies in end-of-life care (Ostherr, Killoran, Shegog, & Bruera, 2016). In most studies, communication technologies were used for multiple purposes, with the most common involving information/education, as a decision aid, and relieving symptom distress. In other research, online communities were particularly important for emotional support among caregivers and family members of patients in hospice (Buis, 2008).

Communication technologies are also important in the delivery of hospice care. Telehospice involves the use of technologies to provide end-of-life care to people in their homes. Videophones as well as other monitoring devices placed in a health provider's office and patients' homes make possible synchronous exchanges with full audio and video. Telehospice visits serve to supplement in-home visits by hospice professionals. In one relatively large study, nurses initiated almost all of the hospice video calls and visits tended to focus on routine follow-ups or physical assessments

(Whitten, Doolittle, & Mackert, 2004). Less than one-third of cases required an additional home visit from a health provider.

Telehospice appears to have several advantages for patients. At the most basic level, telehospice can provide immediate access to health care professionals (Whitten et al., 2004). Their increased access may foster a sense of connection and security with one's health care provider (Maudlin, Keene, & Kobb, 2006). In one study, caregivers of a loved one who was at the end of life reported a statistically significant reduction in anxiety as a result of access to telehospice but no change in quality of life (Demiris, Oliver, Courtney, & Day, 2007). Telehospice technologies can also encourage connections among family members who cannot be physically present (Whitten, Doolittle, Mackert, & Rush, 2003). The potential to overcome distance may be particularly important to patients in rural areas. Although less than half of the patients in one study were from rural sites, they accounted for almost 60 percent of all telehospice visits (Whitten et al., 2004). A few disadvantages for patients have also been identified related to technological concerns (Whitten et al., 2004) and patients' ability and willingness to use the technology as their health or the health of their loved one diminishes (Oliver, Demiris, Day, Courtney, & Porock, 2006).

For providers, telehospice offers time savings stemming from reduced travel, along with the potential for greater involvement with patients and improved care (Day, Demiris, Oliver, Courtney, & Hensel, 2007; Whitten et al., 2003). The video component appears to be particularly important for allowing health providers to better understand patient needs and problems as well as determine whether an in-person visit is necessary (Demiris, Oliver, Fleming, & Edison, 2004; Doolittle et al., 1998; Whitten et al., 2003). Telehospice technologies can also serve as a means to coordinate and facilitate participation among family members, the patient, and health care professionals in making decisions and providing hospice care (Wittenberg-Lyles, Oliver, Demiris, & Baldwin, 2010). Cost savings are a final advantage. Telehospice visits have been shown to be considerably less expensive than traditional in-person home hospice visits (Doolittle, 2000).

In addition to these advantages, several disadvantages of telehospice for providers have been identified. Comfort with the technology (Whitten et al., 2003) and technological problems involving equipment reliability and the quality of audio/video (Day et al., 2007) are potential barriers. Concerns with patients' readiness or ability to use the technology can also present challenges (Demiris et al., 2004). Some hospice providers even saw telehospice as a threat to the nature of their work and, in particular, their autonomy (Whitten, Doolittle, & Mackert, 2005). A final barrier involves organizational support. In at least one study, hospice providers felt that telehospice was not embraced by management and participation was not properly incentivized (Whitten, Holtz, Meyer, & Nazione, 2009).

Coping with and Communicating about the End of Life

Beyond the specific context of hospice and palliative care, communication technologies can play an important role as patients cope with the end of life. In a case study of a 30-year-old man facing terminal cancer, blogging allowed the man to articulate his "considerable existential distress" and evaluate the meaning of his suffering (Lowney & O'Brien, 2012, p. 858). In another study, blogs were used by patients with cancer to leave something behind and be remembered (Chiu & Hsieh, 2013). Blogging was a way for some of the women to leave a record and be remembered. Another motivation for blogging was to confront death. Blogging allowed some women to manage their uncertainty about the possibility of dying. An in-depth analysis of one blogger's experience coping with cancer further underscores the importance of narrative and storytelling at the end of life (Riggs, 2014). The blog served as a mechanism for communal sense-making between the blogger and his readers about the meaning of life and death. In other research, participation in a breast cancer online community helped some members come to terms with their mortality (Williams & Goh, 2015). Members were encouraged to accept their cancer, the possibility of death, and the potential in their circumstances.

Preliminary evidence also indicates that the nature of patients' communication patterns online change as they approach the end of life. In a case study of one women participating in an online breast cancer support intervention, the prevalence of several message types peaked as she entered hospice or just prior to her death (Wen, McTavish, Kreps, Wise, & Gustafson, 2011). Expressions of appreciation for the support community, spiritual expressions, notes about the impact of cancer on her personal relationships, and messages about her own death were all more prevalent at the end of her life. Other research offers insights about the evolution of end-of-life discourse online. In a study of women blogging about cancer, talk about the end of life was prominent after beginning treatment (Keim-Malpass &

Steeves, 2012). Some of the women began coming to terms with the possibility of death. A shift was also observed over time in which the women who wrote about mortality became more comfortable with this topic.

Beyond individual cases, broader trends in online discourse about end-of-life issues have been examined. An analysis of posts to the microblogging platform Twitter over the course of two years showed that almost 700,000 messages contained one of 13 terms related to palliative care (Nwosu, Debattista, Rooney, & Mason, 2015). "End-of-life," "#hpm" (i.e., the hashtag for the hospice and palliative care community), and "palliative care" were the three most common terms. A sentiment analysis showed that almost 90 percent of the posts were more positive than a baseline group of posts made during the same time period. Other researchers have evaluated the content of webpages dedicated to topics such as palliative care (Kozlov & Carpenter, 2015) and suicide (Krysinska & Andriessen, 2010; Westerlund, Hadlaczky, & Wasserman, 2012). An analysis of websites related to suicide conducted during 2005, 2009, and 2012 showed that most information was from institutional sources, focused on research and prevention, and adopted a prevention-focused approach (Westerlund et al., 2012).

Digital Death and Legacy

Communication technologies may continue to play an important role after death. At the present time, questions abound about one's digital estate. Who owns or may access one's personal computer or e-mail? What happens to all of the images, videos, and text one may have shared using social media? Researchers have noted the legal or policy-related difficulties of maintaining or closing a loved one's online accounts, ranging from e-mail to online shopping and social media, after they have died (Locasto, Massimi, & DePasquale, 2011). Indeed, some companies operating social media platforms do not have a provision in their terms of service to terminate the agreement at the time of a user's death (McCallig, 2014). In such cases, information contributed to the site would continue to belong to the company.

At least partially in response to such difficulties, technologies have been proposed and developed that allow users to have greater control over their digital legacy. Two general types of services exists (N. Wright, 2014). Asset maintenance services make it possible for people to control their digital assets after their death. These options entail specifying what should happen if one's account becomes inactive, who should be notified, and the possibility of deleting the account (Prates, Rosson, & de Souza, 2015). Posthumous scheduling services are designed to allow one to schedule and post social media content after one's death.

There has also been some initial movement toward developing technologies that help people construct their digital legacy (Meese, Nansen, Kohn, Arnold, & Gibbs, 2015). One group of researchers, for example, proposed a technology that allows people to save and store memories during their lifetime for the purpose of publishing them after their death (Hall, Bosevski, & Larkin, 2006). The memories would be presented along with the geographic location of where they were created. Another group of researchers focused on "life-logging," which involves cataloging one's personal digital information such as documents, images, videos, and other artifacts in preparation for one's death (Thomas & Briggs, 2014). They conducted focus groups about this activity and reported mixed responses among older adults. Although the potential for family members and others to get to know them better was appealing to some participants, concerns were raised about who could access such information. Similarly mixed responses were reported in a study examining the potential to receive posthumous messages from a loved one (Jamison-Powell et al., 2016). Some participants recognized the possibility that such messages could make it more difficult to cope with grief and cause upset, whereas other respondents reported that, when carefully crafted, they might provide comfort.

To summarize, although the overall volume of research is limited, there is reason to believe that communication technologies have important implications for hospice care, communication about the end of life, and in one's digital legacy. The Internet played a noteworthy role in palliative care patients' efforts to acquire medical information, intraprofessional communication, and in providing support for hospice caregivers and patients' family members. Communication technologies such as blogs served as a mechanism for people facing illness to cope with the end of life and were used in unique ways as they approached death. Growing concerns about what happens to one's digital estate after death has been a topic of concern. Researchers have endeavored to develop technologies that allow people to gain control over their digital remains and manage their digital legacy.

Digital Bereavement and Mourning

In addition to the end of life, communication technologies can play an important role among people who have experienced the death of a loved one. Bereavement, digital memorialization, and grief support are three specific contexts where the implications of communication technologies are particularly significant. Each of these topics will be considered in the following sections.

Communication Technologies and Bereavement

Several communication technologies can be significant during bereavement. Researchers interviewing people who had lost someone close due to suicide found that e-mail offered a less emotionally and physically burdensome means than the telephone or face-to-face communication to inform and update friends and family about the death (Chapple & Ziebland, 2011). E-mail and other technologies have also been touted as useful tools for notifying and coordinating mourners in the process of making funeral arrangements (Moncur et al., 2012). In another study, communication technologies were used to communicate with loved ones after their death (Odom, Harper, Sellen, Kirk, & Banks, 2010). Respondents reported sending e-mail messages, text messages, phone calls, and SNS messages to the deceased. Although this activity declined over time, it served to maintain a connection with the deceased.

Individual technologies, particularly SNSs, also appear to be consequential during bereavement. SNSs have been found to be valuable for learning and sharing information about the deceased (Rossetto, Lannutti, & Strauman, 2015) as well as for interacting with other mourners and allowing grief to extend beyond formal contexts such as funerals and into everyday life (Brubaker, Hayes, & Dourish, 2013). At least one study offered evidence that SNSs can be a site for communal coping (Lingel, 2013). In addition to these advantages, several limitations of SNSs have been identified. Depersonalization was one limitation that occurred when the serious nature of the death was minimized, and another involved misunderstandings about expressions of grief in this context (Rossetto et al., 2015). SNS use may also create challenges for overcoming grief when users unexpectedly encounter the deceased through automated notifications and previously posted images (Brubaker et al., 2013; Odom et al., 2010; Rossetto et al., 2015).

Broader trends in bereavement-related communication technology use have been examined. Researchers analyzing the search logs from America Online over an eight-month period found that searches related to bereavement tended to focus on the social and legal aspects of death rather than on grieving (Ruthven, 2012). The most popular search terms involved rituals and behaviors such as funeral planning. Searches about financial and legal aspects were less common but noteworthy. Less than 10 percent of searches involved the process of grieving. In an analysis of more than 1,000 images posted to an image-sharing SNS along with the hashtag "#funeral," self-portraits or "selfies" were the most common types of images (Gibbs, Meese, Arnold, Nansen, & Carter, 2015). The accompanying labels (i.e., hashtags) revealed a variety of concerns by the photographers, ranging from self-presentation to self-reflection. Images of family were also common along with photos capturing funeral rituals. These studies underscore the social nature of grieving and bereavement rituals.

Some researchers have suggested that technology design can help facilitate bereavement (Gray & Coulton, 2013). They advocated designing technologies that recognize varying cultural values about death and support the novel practices developed by users. One SNS developed specifically for bereavement support was used relatively infrequently by study participants (Massimi, 2013). Interviews revealed that, although participants were in need of support, using the SNS required a great deal of emotional effort. Participants felt compelled to engage in "grief work" on the site, which made using it a chore.

Digital Memorialization and Mourning

Communication technologies are particularly conspicuous during mourning, which involves cultural rituals that serve as public displays of grief (Cowles & Rodgers, 1991). Researchers have identified at least three types of online memorials (Roberts, 2012). "Web cemeteries" are websites dedicated solely to memorializing the dead, whereas webring memorials involve personal webpages joined together for the purpose of memorializing one or more people. The third category includes memorialized accounts and pages on SNS platforms. All three types of memorials are similar in that a unique page or website is dedicated to an individual who has died and readers are able to contribute comments.

Online memorials are fairly pervasive. More than half of the young adults surveyed in one study had visited the SNS page for someone who was deceased, and more than one third had joined a group dedicated to someone who had died (Carroll & Landry, 2010). Additionally, content analyses tend to show that fairly diverse demographic and social groups have been memorialized. Memorials on websites (Roberts & Vidal, 2000) and SNSs (Kern, Forman, & Gil-Egui, 2013) were dedicated to people across the age spectrum at the time of their death. Yet some groups appear more frequently than others. Memorials dedicated to males were more common than females on websites (Roberts & Vidal, 2000) and SNSs (Kern et al., 2013). Notably, a substantial number of the memorials examined in two studies were dedicated to people who had died suddenly or violently (Kern et al., 2013; Roberts & Vidal, 2000).

Memorials tend to be created by a friend or family member of the deceased (Krysinska & Andriessen, 2015). Almost three-quarters of the memorials examined in two studies were constructed within five years of the deceased's death (Krysinska & Andriessen, 2015; Roberts & Vidal, 2000). It was not uncommon, however, for memorials to be created 10 years or more after death (Krysinska & Andriessen, 2015; Roberts & Vidal, 2000). Entries on memorial websites averaged between approximately 100 and 200 words (Roberts & Vidal, 2000), and contributions to SNS memorials averaged approximately 40 words (Getty et al., 2011). Posts to SNS memorials after death contained a greater proportion of words related to grief and social relationships than posts made before the person had died.

A broad coalition of people—including those who were acquaintances or did not personally know the deceased—contribute to online memorials. Although an analysis of memorials dedicated to suicide victims indicated that most comments were authored by immediate family members (Krysinska & Andriessen, 2015), several studies of SNS memorials have shown that people who did not have a close relationship with the deceased were also contributors (DeGroot, 2014; Marwick & Ellison, 2012; Williams & Merten, 2009). These results are consistent with the findings from a survey of young adults in which more than half of the sample reported that at least one connection in their SNS network was deceased (Egnoto, Sirianni, Ortega, & Stefanone, 2014). Two-thirds of the deceased were acquaintances, and one-quarter of the respondents reported engaging in some type of grieving behavior on the SNS after they discovered the death. People who are not close with the deceased appear to contribute to online memorials because they identify with the deceased in some way (DeGroot, 2014). This may involve being an acquaintance of the deceased (e.g., clerk at a store where he or she frequently shopped), having a network connection (e.g., aunt's best friend), witnessing the deceased's death, or sharing a key similarity with the deceased (e.g., victim of a specific crime).

Five primary themes have been identified in the content of online memorials. First, like traditional eulogies, messages posted in online memorials may chronical the lives of the deceased (Hume & Bressers, 2009; Krysinska & Andriessen, 2015; Roberts & Vidal, 2000). Commenters may post stories about the deceased and/or discuss the deceased's beliefs and values (Carroll & Landry, 2010). Praise for the deceased was noted in several studies (Carroll & Landry, 2010; Marwick & Ellison, 2012). Negative comments about the deceased have also been identified on SNSs (Leonard & Toller, 2012) and memorials posted on video-sharing websites (Gibson & Altena, 2014), although they were typically refuted in one study of SNS memorials (Marwick & Ellison, 2012).

A second theme involves condolences and messages to family members (DeGroot, 2014; Hume & Bressers, 2009; Leonard & Toller, 2012). Online memorials were used to recognize and show support for the deceased and the deceased's family. More than two-thirds of the comments in one study contained formulaic condolence phrases such as "RIP" (Klastrup, 2015). Requests for help or guidance from the deceased represent a third theme in online memorial messages. In several studies, commenters to SNS memorials left messages requesting protection or guidance from the deceased (Carroll & Landry, 2010; DeGroot, 2012; Irwin, 2015). Requests were made for the deceased to visit in one's dreams or to look after a family member or pet who also was deceased (DeGroot, 2012).

A fourth theme in messages to the deceased involves explanations for his or her death or otherwise addresses the context of his or her death (Roberts & Vidal, 2000). Such messages were observed in analyses of SNS memorial pages for people who died from suicide (Krysinska & Andriessen, 2015; Leonard & Toller, 2012) and accidents (Klastrup, 2015). These types of comments ranged from justifying the deceased's death to offering insights about how or why the death occurred. In a study of SNS memorials dedicated to everyday people whose dramatic death received significant media attention, comments focused on the way in which people died (Klastrup, 2015). One researcher even found comments from people who witnessed the deceased's death (DeGroot, 2014).

Finally, philosophizing about the meaning of life or spirituality was a theme in online memorials (DeGroot, 2012). One group of researchers found messages related to religion or spirituality in just over 10 percent of the contributions they examined from memorial websites (Krysinska, Andriessen, & Corveleyn, 2014). These messages addressed topics such as God's will, peace for the deceased, and the afterlife. Another group found excerpts from religious verse in the memorials they examined (Roberts & Vidal, 2000). Table 7.2 illustrates each of the five themes.

Online memorials serve two functions for mourners making contributions (DeGroot, 2012). First, contributions to online memorials can help mourners to understand loss. The sense-making function of online memorials can be observed in the language used by contributors. Expressions of emotion have been identified in several analyses (DeGroot, 2014; Hume & Bressers, 2009; Krysinska & Andriessen, 2015). In addition to negative emotions such as sadness, grief, anger, and guilt (Carroll & Landry, 2010; Krysinska & Andriessen, 2015; Williams & Merten, 2009), expressions of love and other positive emotions have also been reported (Krysinska & Andriessen, 2015). Expressing emotions is an important part of the grieving process that may facilitate mourners' efforts to come to terms with the death. Expressing one's feeling about loss could be a means through which that loss may be better understood.

The second function of online memorials for mourners involves continuing connections with the deceased (DeGroot, 2012). This function is evident in the language used in online memorials. In an analysis of posts made to the SNS memorials, language reflecting psychological distance was greater before than after death (Getty et al., 2011). Other researchers

Table 7.2

Themes in Online Memorials

Theme	Definition
Biographizing	Messages describing the deceased's behavior, beliefs, and values.
Condolences	Messages expressing well wishes for the family and friends of the deceased.
Requests	Messages asking the deceased for help or guidance.
Explanations	Messages describing or justifying the deceased's death.
Philosophizing	Messages considering the meaning of life or spirituality.

reported a tendency for mourners to write as if the deceased were present (Kern et al., 2013; Klastrup, 2015; Williams & Merten, 2009). Memorial contributions were written directly to the deceased as if he or she could read them and respond. Although this pattern was less evident in research on memorial websites conducted during the late 1990s, almost one-third of the memorial messages in one study were directed to the deceased (Roberts & Vidal, 2000). Writing directly to the deceased—as opposed to about him or her—is important because it suggests that online memorials are being used to converse with the deceased and sustain one's relationship.

A final aspect of language use by mourners in online memorials that merits noting involves the audience that is assumed or targeted in mourners' messages. Online memorials are public, in that one's contributions are visible to others who are presumably mourning the loss of the same person. Although early research examining memorial websites showed that contributions frequently addressed or were written for the audience as one might find in a traditional eulogy (Roberts & Vidal, 2000), more recent studies have suggested that references to the community of mourners were relatively uncommon (Church, 2013)—with the exception of sharing condolences with the family (Klastrup, 2015). This finding is significant because an important function of eulogies is to restore community among survivors (Church, 2013). Online memorials appear to be unique from other rhetorical genres of memorialization, in that grief is shared in view of others but not necessarily communally.

Grief Support Online

In addition to online memorials, communication technologies have had significant implications for grief-related social support. In coping with grief after the loss of a loved one, social support can be a critical resource. Online communities are one important site for acquiring grief support, with respondents in one study indicating that they spent just over seven hours per week online for this purpose (van der Houwen, Stroebe, Schut, Stroebe, & van den Bout, 2010). Other researchers have noted the potential of SNSs for receiving grief support (Brubaker et al., 2013; Rossetto et al., 2015).

A lack of offline support is one reason for seeking grief support online. Just over 10 percent of all posts made to three online grief communities reflected insufficient or inadequate support offline (Döveling, 2015). In an online community dedicated to mothers who had experienced the loss of an unborn child, some women described their husbands or partners as emotionally distant and disconnected from their grief (Capitulo, 2004). In another study, current online community users reported lower levels of support available from family and friends, greater levels of grief, and greater levels of emotional loneliness than did former members (van der Houwen et al., 2010).

Several advantages of online bereavement support have been identified. One important advantage of SNSs for support involves the volume of messages received offering condolences. Focus groups with bereaved young adults revealed that receiving a large quantity of messages led the young adults to feel cared for and loved (Wandel, 2009). The fact that the condolences came from a diverse cross-section of their social network (e.g., family members, acquaintances, etc.) was also meaningful. Another advantage of SNSs concerns witnessing the grief of others (Rossetto et al., 2015). Knowing that others were grieving and learning about what the deceased meant to others can foster feelings of community and a sense of solidarity in coping with loss. Other advantages of online communities include the potential to remain anonymous and the availability of potential support providers (Chapple & Ziebland, 2011).

In addition to the advantages, researchers have reported some disadvantages of SNSs for grief support (Rossetto et al., 2015; Wandel, 2009). One major disadvantage concerns the potential to be overwhelmed by the volume of condolence messages. Feeling compelled to respond to well-wishers can be taxing. Problems with "bandwagon mourners" who are perceived to be insincere and concerns with privacy are other disadvantages. A final disadvantage involves members of one's social network using the SNS to avoid face-to-face contact with the bereaved. Limitations of online support communities include the potential for upset caused by reading others' accounts and the amount of time spent participating in the community (Chapple & Ziebland, 2011).

Research examining the nature of communication within online grief support communities offers several additional insights. A content analysis of a listserv used by mothers who had experienced the loss of an unborn child revealed that transformation or metamorphosis was a key theme in the group's discourse (Capitulo, 2004). The group was a means for members to transform their identity to that of the "mommy of an angel," and angels were an important symbol for the group. Self-disclosure played a key role in support-provision attempts in another study of online bereavement support communities (Swartwood, Veach, Kuhne, Lee, & Ji, 2011). Community members responded to an initial contribution from a fellow member by sharing their own experiences. These disclosures tended to acknowledge the original poster's loss, linked that loss with their own experiences, and then provided advice or comfort. The validation of grief was also an important function of the community. Members normalized grief and gave others permission to grieve, which served to offset the stigma sometimes associated with grieving.

In other research, a small group of bereaved former caregivers was given access to a private SNS group to discuss their efforts in coping with grief over the course of nine months (Wittenberg-Lyles et al., 2015). Most of the comments made to the group concerned members' efforts to cope with restoration-oriented stressors involving difficulties remaking one's life in absence of the deceased. Other members offered emotional support and advice regarding challenging tasks related to restoration, discussed coping strategies, and shared turning points in their own bereavement. Discussion of loss-oriented stressors was less common but still prevalent. Loss-oriented stressors involved difficulties related to their loved one's death or absence. Members discussed ways to manage anticipated and unanticipated triggers that served to remind them of their loss.

Although research examining the outcomes of using communication technologies for grief support is limited, some evidence suggests that it can be beneficial. In a survey of active grief support community members, almost half agreed that their participation in the community made their grief less severe (Hartig & Viola, 2016). Respondents who had been a community member for more than a year reported significantly less grief severity than community members who had participated for less than one year. Among three online bereavement communities popular in Germany, researchers found that longer conversation threads were more likely to include discussions of issues beyond bereavement (Döveling, 2015). The researchers argued that this finding offers evidence that online support communities allowed the bereaved to ultimately move beyond their loss and return to their everyday lives. In contrast to the preceding findings, a survey of online support community members showed no change in the mental well-being of active users relative to nonusers over three time points (van der Houwen et al., 2010).

Taken together, research examining digital bereavement and mourning suggests that communication technologies have several important implications. Various communication technologies such as e-mail and social media appear to be valuable for information sharing and coordination after the death of a family member or friend. Digital memorials have become a prominent cite for mourning. Memorials serve as a means to make sense of loss and maintain connections with the deceased. Communication technologies have also been used for grief support. Several advantages and disadvantages exist for using technologies such as online communities and SNSs for coping with grief after the loss of a loved one.

Issues Warranting Additional Attention in Research on the End of Life

The body of research examining the implications of communication technologies at the end of life and bereavement is still in its infancy. Although existing research has significantly advanced our understanding of those topics, significant work remains. Three general issues warrant greater consideration.

First, it is critical to dedicate additional efforts to explore the implications of communication technologies in hospice care. The uses and effects of communication technologies among hospice providers are valuable topics to consider. In addition to examining intraprofessional coordination, it is important to investigate how health providers use communication technologies to share information with patients and their families. Hospice care often involves a number of stakeholders beyond physicians and patients, and communication technologies can and likely do play a critical role in coordinating information and care. Additionally, it is important to further examine the role of communication technologies in end-of-life decision making. Communication technologies may be critical for acquiring information and navigating the uncertainty associated with end-of-life care decisions.

A second issue that merits additional attention involves the outcomes of online mourning and bereavement. Although researchers have endeavored to better understand the content of online memorials, more needs to be known about their effects on bereavement processes. It would be worthwhile to investigate how and why participating in online memorials impacts efforts at coping with loss. The consequences of online memorials for broader societal perceptions of death and dying also are important to understand. Given data showing that many SNS users have a connection or "friend" on the site who is deceased (Carroll & Landry, 2010), it seems possible that this exposure to death may influence societal perceptions of death and dying. Similarly, it would be worthwhile to explore the consequences of documenting end-of-life experiences for the family and friends of the deceased. Women blogging about their cancer experiences noted that a motivation for blogging was to leave something behind for their children to know them better (Chiu & Hsieh, 2013). Exploring the effects of such efforts on families would be valuable.

A third and final set of issues that desire greater attention involve how communication technologies might be used to foster a more peaceful and dignified death. Communication technologies could be used to support sense-making at the end of life. They might be incorporated into decision aids and help facilitate end-of-life decision making. Communication technologies may be valuable in connecting and promoting closure among members of patients' social networks at the end of life. As these examples illustrate, research would be valuable to further explore the potential of communication technologies for ensuring that people are able to die gracefully and feel confident about their legacy.

Conclusion

The potential implications of communication technologies at the end of life and bereavement are just beginning to be realized. Telehospice might be able to expand and perhaps even improve hospice care. Blogs and online communities appear to offer opportunities for making sense of death and leaving something behind for loved ones. These technologies, along with SNSs, can assist the bereaved in coping with their loss and memorializing their loved ones who have died. Yet questions remain about the ways in which communication technologies can be used to promote a more peaceful death along with one's digital remains and legacy. Further exploration of these and related issues is critical to better understand the uses and effects of communication technologies among those facing the end of life or loss of a loved one. Such efforts will ultimately help to advance our state of knowledge about coping with illness digitally.

8 Model of Digital Coping with Illness

Communication technologies can play a central role in the process of coping with illness. Indeed, the preceding chapters illustrate the myriad of coping functions enabled by communication technologies. Patients used the Internet to seek information prior to visiting a health care provider (Thomson, Siminoff, & Longo, 2012) and after their consultation (Bell, Hu, Orrange, & Kravitz, 2011; Li, Orrange, Kravitz, & Bell, 2014). Online communities offered a means to manage negative emotions (Shim, Cappella, & Han, 2011) and offset support deficits in offline relationships (Chung, 2013). Blogs allowed patients to make sense of their illness experience (Rains & Keating, 2015) and cogitate about existential concerns (Chiu & Hsieh, 2013). Social network sites (SNSs) functioned as a tool for constructing (Krysinska & Andriessen, 2015) and protecting (Marwick & Ellison, 2012) the legacy of a deceased loved one. E-mail enabled patients to receive emotional support from health care providers (Turner et al., 2013), and videophones allowed patients at the end of life to acquire advice and feedback from a hospice nurse (Whitten, Doolittle, & Mackert, 2004). In each of the preceding examples, communication technologies were used to perform specific coping activities and manage particular forms of distress stemming from illness.

Despite the potential importance of communication technologies in coping with illness, the body of scholarship on this topic remains largely disconnected. Researchers tend to focus on a single issue such as information seeking or technology such as blogs without considering other activities or technologies. Relatively few attempts have been made to identify factors that transcend digital coping. The cumulative result of this trend is that we know a fair amount about the implications of specific communication technologies in distinct contexts, but we lack an understanding of how those parts fit together into a broader whole. There remains a critical need to consolidate our existing knowledge and develop a general model explaining the role of communication technologies in coping with illness.

The central objective of this chapter is to outline a model of digital coping. The model explains how communication technologies may be used systematically in coping efforts. It advances our understanding of the role played by communication technologies in coping with illness in at least two important ways. First, elements of illness and communication technologies that are central to digital coping are identified. The most salient forms of distress, affordances of communication technologies, and activities of digital coping are explained. Second, the ways in which these components contribute to digital coping efforts are described. Digital coping is considered as a process in which forms of distress and communication technology affordances contribute to specific coping behaviors.

The remainder of this chapter serves to detail the model of digital coping. The assumptions of the model are first described, followed by a discussion of the major components and functions. The implications of the model for researchers and health care professionals are then considered to conclude the chapter.

Model Foundations and Assumptions

The digital coping model developed in this chapter is rooted in broader ideas about the functions of stress and coping developed by Lazarus and associates (Lazarus, 1966, 2012; Lazarus & Folkman, 1984). Their transactional model of stress and coping details the process by which people respond to stressors and has played a prominent role in coping research throughout the past five decades (Wethington, Glanz, & Schwartz, 2015). The transactional model involves two general steps. First, people assess the meaning of an event. Primary appraisals involve evaluating the relevance and importance of an event, whereas secondary appraisals focus on one's ability to respond to the event. These two appraisals in conjunction provide an evaluation of the stressor and what might be done about it.

The second step in responding to a stressor involves coping efforts enacted to address the stressor. Although many specific actions are possible, there are two general classes of coping responses. Problem-focused coping centers on changing the environment to mitigate the stressor. This response could involve taking action to directly address the source of distress (e.g., taking medication to combat physical pain). Emotion-focused coping involves changing one's reaction to or perspective of the stressor. This response might include trying to see the stressor in a different light (e.g., coming to see pain as an integral part of the healing process). Different activities may serve as problem- or emotion-focused coping, and these two types of coping may co-occur. In the transactional model of stress and coping, it is not assumed that coping activities will necessarily be objectively helpful or beneficial. It is possible that coping may fail to address the immediate stressor or even result in additional problems or deleterious long-term consequences.

An example would be useful to illustrate the stress and coping process. A patient with prostate cancer experiencing acute fatigue may first appraise the relevance of the fatigue and its meaning. One possible primary appraisal is that the fatigue is a serious concern because it indicates that one's health is declining. This evaluation is followed by a secondary appraisal of the patient's options for addressing the fatigue or its meaning. In this case, the patient might consider whether the fatigue could be managed or reversed. Primary and secondary appraisals can prompt a coping response. The patient with prostate cancer may consult a doctor in hopes of identifying a remedy for the fatigue (i.e., problem-focused coping) or vent his frustrations about the fatigue in a prostate cancer online community (i.e., emotion-focused coping). These activities may range in effectiveness.

With background information about stress and coping in place, it is important to discuss two key assumptions that ground the digital coping model. One is that communication technologies can play an important role in coping with illness. The various affordances of communication technologies offer novel opportunities for coping. Communication technologies can be used to engage in a range of coping activities in response to specific forms of distress. As such, the digital coping model detailed in this chapter builds from prior research on stress and coping but privileges the role of communication technologies. Appraisal and coping are considered specifically in the context of communication technology use. This approach may overlook or minimize some factors that appear in other stress-coping research. Yet it is critical to isolate the implications of communication technologies in coping with illness. The significance of illness and the central role of communication technologies in contemporary society warrant such an approach. Moreover, because it shares the same basic framework, the model developed in this chapter is compatible with Lazarus and colleagues' (Lazarus, 1966, 2012; Lazarus & Folkman, 1984) transactional model of stress and coping.

A second assumption that serves to ground the model developed in this chapter involves the approach used in considering communication technologies. The model does not isolate any single communication technology such as e-mail, blogs, or SNSs. Instead, it is focused on those affordances that transcend individual technologies. Affordances involve the broader opportunities for action that technologies are perceived to enable (Gibson, 1977; Markus & Silver, 2008; Norman, 1999). Given the rapid development and diffusion of new communication technologies during the past few decades, focusing on individual technologies would likely yield a model that would rapidly become obsolete. Considering affordances offers a robust strategy to ensure that the model is applicable to contemporary technologies as well as those developed in the future. Although research on individual technologies is discussed in presenting the model, it is included simply to illustrate the broader affordances or coping activities.

Digital Coping Model

Building on Lazarus and colleagues' (Lazarus, 1966, 2012; Lazarus & Folkman, 1984) work on stress and coping, the digital coping model has been developed to explicate the role of communication technologies in the process of coping with illness. The central purpose of the model is to explain how and why people facing serious illness use technologies as a coping resource. Appraisals and subsequent coping efforts are considered in the context of communication technology use specifically among people facing illness. Primary appraisals are conceptualized in terms of five sources of distress that were prominent throughout the research reviewed in the preceding chapters. Secondary appraisals involve evaluating one or more of seven key communication technology affordances. Situational and individual difference factors that may contribute to the salience of particular affordances are also identified. Together, the sources of distress and affordances are proposed to shape coping efforts. Five specific lines of coping enacted

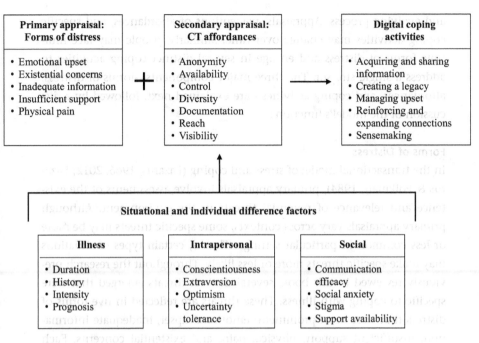

Primary appraisal: Forms of distress	Secondary appraisal: CT affordances	Digital coping activities
• Emotional upset • Existential concerns • Inadequate information • Insufficient support • Physical pain	• Anonymity • Availability • Control • Diversity • Documentation • Reach • Visibility	• Acquiring and sharing information • Creating a legacy • Managing upset • Reinforcing and expanding connections • Sensemaking

Situational and individual difference factors

Illness	Intrapersonal	Social
• Duration • History • Intensity • Prognosis	• Conscientiousness • Extraversion • Optimism • Uncertainty tolerance	• Communication efficacy • Social anxiety • Stigma • Support availability

Figure 8.1
Digital Coping Model

using communication technologies are discussed. The model is illustrated in figure 8.1.

Prior to detailing the components of the digital coping model, it is important to consider a few caveats. First, the model has been developed in an effort to bring order to existing research and explain the key factors involved in digital coping. The model is primarily intended to be descriptive. However, several specific predictions are discussed in considering the functions of the model. These predictions are intended to be representative and not exhaustive. Other predictions may be possible. A second and related caveat involves the outcomes of digital coping activities. The efficacy of the various activities is not assumed in the model. Any one of the coping activities may lead to outcomes that might be objectively deemed therapeutic or detrimental. Potential positive and negative consequences are briefly considered, along with each coping activity. Finally, in an effort to detail the individual components of digital coping, the model is presented in a static manner. However, coping is assumed to be a dynamic and evolving process. Appraisals, perceptions of affordances, and specific coping activities may change over time. Similarly, people may face multiple forms of distress and engage in several distinct coping activities to address a single stressor. The three major components—forms of distress, affordances, and coping activities—are explained next, followed by a discussion of the model's functions.

Forms of Distress

In the transactional model of stress and coping (Lazarus, 1966, 2012; Lazarus & Folkman, 1984), primary appraisals involve assessments of the existence and relevance of potential threats in the environment. Although primary appraisals vary across contexts, some specific threats may be more or less common in particular settings. That is, certain types of situations may make specific threats more or less likely. Throughout the research previously reviewed in this book, several distinct threats emerged that were specific to coping with illness. These threats are reflected in five forms of distress that were most prominent: emotional upset, inadequate information, insufficient support, physical pain, and existential concerns. Each form of distress represents a unique potential threat faced by people coping with illness.

Emotional Upset   Perhaps the most common form of distress identified in the research reviewed in this book is emotional upset. Although it may take several forms, emotional upset was routinely experienced throughout the preceding chapters as negative emotions (Bar-Lev, 2008; Lieberman & Goldstein, 2006; Marcus, Westra, Eastwood, & Barnes, 2012; Owen et al., 2005). Sadness, anger, and fear were common, along with related emotions such as shame and hopelessness. Negative emotions stemmed from a myriad of sources related to experiencing illness. Beyond specific emotions, upset can be observed in other aversive states such as frustration or a more general sense of discontentment. Emotional upset is a potentially significant and pervasive form of distress among patients.

Inadequate Information   Perceptions of unsatisfactory or inadequate information is another form of distress evident in the preceding chapters (Balka, Krueger, Holmes, & Stephen, 2010; Dolce, 2011; Kirschning & von Kardorff, 2008; Markle, Attell, & Treiber, 2015). Inadequate information involves uncertainty or a lack of knowledge about a particular topic related to illness. It may result from novel symptoms, conflicting recommendations, confusing medical jargon, limited interaction time with health providers, questions about illness prognosis, or any number of other sources. Inadequate information leaves patients unable to satisfactorily understand their illness or illness-related experiences.

Insufficient Support   An insufficient support network is a third form of distress that was salient in the preceding chapters. It can take the form of the absence of support providers or the presence of ineffective providers. Inadequate support from family and friends resulted from the inability to fully grasp patients' circumstances (Malik & Coulson, 2008; Rodham, McCabe, & Blake, 2009). Family and friends had difficulty understanding the nuances or magnitude of the challenges that patients faced. Patients also reported a more general sense of social isolation (Hinton, Kurinczuk, & Ziebland, 2010; Ressler, Bradshaw, Gualtieri, & Chui, 2012). They felt set apart from others who were not ill or otherwise alone in experiencing their specific health condition.

Physical Pain   The physical discomfort associated with illness is another form of distress evident in the preceding chapters. It can stem from the nature of illness or specific treatment regimens and may be chronic or acute. The immediate discomfort associated with pain can tax one's well-being. It may create difficulties accomplishing daily activities, maintaining personal relationships, and a plethora of other specific challenges (Keim-Malpass & Steeves, 2012; Radin, 2006; Rodham et al., 2009). In these ways, physical pain can be a significant source of distress among patients.

Existential Concerns   A final form of distress evident in the previous chapters involves existential concerns. Serious illness can serve to raise questions about the meaning of life and one's place in the world. Some patients may consider their mortality (Williams & Goh, 2015) or question the reason for their suffering (Mirivel & Thombre, 2010). Existential concerns also can be reflected in patients' desire to integrate chronic illness into their everyday lives (Liu, Inkpen, & Pratt, 2015; Markle et al., 2015). Patients may wish to regain a sense of normalcy or construct a new or revised identity that accounts for illness. Such existential worries are a final form of distress relevant to patients.

Communication Technology Affordances
In the transactional model of stress and coping (Lazarus, 1966, 2012; Lazarus & Folkman, 1984), secondary appraisals involve considering one's potential to deal with a stressor. They focus on one's ability and the resources available to manage the stressor or its consequences. In the digital coping model, the implications of communication technologies for coping are privileged. Secondary appraisals take the form of considering the affordances of communication technologies.

An affordance is unique from the features of a technology and involves the way that the technology is perceived and used (Gibson, 1977; Markus & Silver, 2008; Norman, 1999). Although technological features contribute to affordances, affordances are distinct in that they are firmly rooted in users' perceptions about the types of activity a technology may support. For example, a feature of e-mail, blogs, online communities, and other technologies is that interactions tend to be text-based and take the form of written language. Perceiving these text-based technologies as a means to document one's interactions with the aim of referring to them in the future would be an affordance. This documentation affordance involves capitalizing on the opportunities provided by text-based technologies to archive one's interactions for future use.

In the preceding chapters of this book, affordances of communication technologies unique to each coping context were identified. Across those contexts, several themes emerged. The following seven affordances represent the salient dimensions of communication technologies in coping with illness: visibility, availability, control, documentation, anonymity, diversity, and reach. Each of the seven affordances will be reviewed in the following paragraphs.

Visibility Visibility involves the potential to observe others and to be observed. This may include witnessing others engage in interactions or gaining access to information they have shared. Members of health-focused online communities noted the value in being able to read about the problems faced by others and the feedback they received from group members (Malik & Coulson, 2008).Visibility also extends to making one's own thoughts and behaviors observable. Blogging served as a means for patients to make friends and family members aware of developments (McCosker & Darcy, 2013) and turn coping into a collaborative endeavor with others facing similar health concerns (Leggatt-Cook & Chamberlain, 2012). In these ways, communication technologies can provide the opportunity to make oneself visible or observe others.

Availability Availability concerns the accessibility of potential coping resources such as people and information. It involves being able to locate resources when they are most needed or desired. Although health information historically has been restricted to people with formal medical training, the Internet has allowed the lay public to access vast quantities of information on demand. One benefit—as well as one challenge—of using the Internet to acquire health information cited by patients is the sheer volume of information available online (Lee, Hoti, Hughes, & Emmerton, 2014). The potential to contact providers outside of traditional office hours was identified as a key advantage of having e-mail access to a health provider (Andreassen, Trondsen, Kummervold, Gammon, & Hjortdahl, 2006; Rosen & Kwoh, 2007). Telemedicine was similarly touted for providing patients immediate access to palliative care (Whitten et al., 2004). Communication technologies can enable or extend access to potential coping resources.

Control Whereas availability concerns the potential to conveniently or immediately access resources, control involves the nature of interaction with those resources. Control refers to one's potential to manage aspects of interaction. The term "interaction" is defined broadly to include communicating with other humans as well as information and computer programs. Control can be influenced by the relative presence of social cues (e.g., nonverbal behaviors), (a)synchrony, contextual norms for behavior, and/or several other factors. Some online community members cited the asynchronous nature of these technologies as an important reason they felt comfortable expressing their thoughts and feelings (Burke, Kraut, & Williams, 2010). The potential to take their time in constructing messages and the ability to edit those messages before sharing them can allow patients to better communicate their ideas. In research on health information seeking, one benefit of Internet use reported by patients involved control over the duration and depth of their information-seeking efforts (Jones et al., 2014). Unlike a medical consultation with a health provider, Internet users can spend as much time and address as many topics as they desire. As these examples illustrate, communication technologies can make it possible for patients to regulate specific features of interaction.

Documentation   Documentation concerns the potential to leave a record of one's interaction or transaction. Records may take the form of audio, video, text, or some combination. Documentation can function to provide a lasting archive that could be consulted in the future. Health bloggers cited the importance of creating a record of their experiences that others facing similar challenges might consult (Sundar, Edwards, Hu, & Stavrositu, 2007) as well as to be accountable for their health goals (Sanford, 2010). In research on patient-provider interaction, e-mail was seen by some providers as being better than the telephone for archiving interactions with patients (Patt, Houston, Jenckes, Sands, & Ford, 2003). Online memorials served to permanently chronical the life of the deceased (Roberts & Vidal, 2000). Communication technologies can make it possible to leave tangible traces of previous interactions or transactions.

Anonymity   Anonymity involves the potential to conceal or shield one's identity while engaging in coping efforts. It is rooted in the perception that one's words or actions cannot be linked with one's legal identity. Anonymity can allow patients to feel more comfortable by mitigating concerns about embarrassment or retribution. It facilitated coping efforts among health bloggers (Rains, 2014), online support community members (Malik & Coulson, 2008; Tanis, 2008a), and people seeking health information online (Rains & Ruppel, 2016). Communication technologies can make it possible for patients to act without disclosing their legal name or other identifying information.

Diversity   Diversity pertains to the types of resources to which patients have access. A primary distinction involves the degree to which communication technologies make it possible to connect with information sources that offer technical or experiential perspectives about illness. Whereas technical perspectives involve medical aspects of illness, experiential perspectives reflect patients' first-hand experiences (Fergie, Hilton, & Hunt, 2016; Kim, Shah, Namkoong, McTavish, & Gustafson, 2013). Diversity is greater when communication technologies make it possible to access more of these two types of content. Research examining health information seeking online has shown that patients desired medical information related to the etiology and treatment of illness (Colombo et al., 2014; Kirschning & von Kardorff, 2008) as well as other patients' unique experiences coping with a given illness (Balka et al., 2010; Paolino et al., 2015). Online community members highlighted the benefits of community participation for learning about medical aspects of an illness as well as other patients' coping strategies (Holbrey & Colson, 2013). Communication technologies can make it possible to connect with diverse coping resources.

Reach   Reach involves the nature of people or information that may be located using a communication technology. It concerns the potential to identify or communicate with a particular person, group, or piece of information. A central benefit of participating in online health communities involved the opportunity to interact with people who have similar health experiences (Holbrey & Colson, 2013; Yli-Uotila, Rantanen, & Suominen, 2014). Caregivers and loved ones of patients at the end of life (Ferguson, Massimi, Crist, & Moffatt, 2014) or who recently died (Moncur, Bikker, Kasket, & Troyer, 2012) cited the importance of being able to share a single message with a large group of people simultaneously. Avoiding the demand to repeat the same message numerous times to different people helped to alleviate some of their stress. Communication technologies can make it possible to connect with specific groups of people or pieces of information.

Coping Activities

In the transactional model of stress and coping (Lazarus, 1966, 2012; Lazarus & Folkman, 1984), coping involves efforts to manage demands that are perceived to exceed one's resources. It includes specific lines of behavior intended to address one or more stressors. Although several general classes of strategies have been identified (Carver, Scheier, & Weintraub, 1989; Folkman & Lazarus, 1980, 1985; Skinner, Edge, Altman, & Sherwood, 2003), the coping responses considered in the digital coping model are uniquely tailored to the context of communication technology use among patients. They are derived from the research reviewed in the previous chapters and include the following five activities: sense-making, managing upset, acquiring and sharing information, reinforcing and expanding connections, and creating a legacy. Each of these activities functions to address one or more forms of distress and can be used in the service of problem- or emotion-focused coping.

As in Lazarus and colleagues' (Lazarus, 1966, 2012; Lazarus & Folkman, 1984) model, it should not be assumed that any coping activity is objectively (un)helpful. The outcome of any digital coping activity is contingent on patients and their broader circumstances. After first describing each coping activity, its potential benefits and limitations will be considered.

Sense-Making One potential response to a stressor is to evaluate its meaning. Sense-making involves the process of drawing connections and structuring one's experiences. Throughout the previous chapters, communication technologies were routinely used for sense-making. Health bloggers reported attempting to organize and better understand their illness-related experiences (Ressler et al., 2012). Sense-making was also reflected in specific forms of language used among health bloggers (Rains & Keating, 2015) and online community members (Shaw, Hawkins, McTavish, Pingree, & Gustafson, 2006). Online memorials were used to comprehend the loss of a loved one (DeGroot, 2012). As these examples illustrate, communication technologies can facilitate efforts to organize and understand the significance of one's experiences.

As a coping strategy, sense-making has potential benefits as well as limitations for patients. Developing a better understanding of one's experiences may lead patients to accept or reappraise their circumstances (Park, 2010; Park & Folkman, 1997). It can help patients gain insight about what is happening to them and what it means for their lives. Yet the increased attention to a source of distress that accompanies sense-making can in some circumstances lead to rumination (Nolen-Hoeksema, McBride, & Larson, 1997). Patients may become overly focused on their concerns, which can serve to exacerbate their distress.

Managing Upset A second form of coping involves attempting to address upset. Although it can take different forms, upset is commonly observed in negative emotions including, but not limited to, anger, sadness, fear, and grief. Managing upset includes efforts to deal with such emotions or their consequences. Attempting to acquire health information online was a way to mitigate the anxiety faced by parents (De Rouck & Leys, 2013). Online communities (van der Houwen, Stroebe, Schut, Stroebe, & van den

Bout, 2010) and SNSs (Rossetto, Lannutti, & Strauman, 2015) have both been identified as important sites for coping with grief. Blogs served as a mechanism for people facing eating disorders to vent anger and frustration (Yeshua-Katz & Martins, 2013) and patients with cancer to manage their emotions (Chung & Kim, 2008). Communication technologies can be used to respond to negative emotions stemming from illness.

Several activities can be used to manage upset. Emotional processing and emotional expression are two specific coping activities that involve directly engaging aversive emotions (Stanton et al., 2000; Stanton, Danoff-Burg, Cameron, & Ellis, 1994). Emotional processing focuses on attempting to understand what one is feeling, whereas emotional expression concerns voicing one's feelings. Each of these activities has the potential to mitigate distress. Talking about or better understanding aversive emotions can— at least temporarily—help to assuage these emotions or their deleterious effects. As with sense-making, however, attempts to manage upset can also result in rumination.

Acquiring and Sharing Information   Although information seeking may function in conjunction with other coping activities such as sense-making and managing upset, it can also be an end in itself. Information can be acquired or shared to address a perceived deficit in one's knowledge or to gain additional knowledge. Physician review websites were used to learn more about and evaluate potential health providers (Thackeray, Crookston, & West, 2013). E-mail was a means for patients to ask their doctors routine questions (Ruiz, García, & Riquelme, 2014). By virtue of participating in an online community, members were routinely exposed to information about their health condition (Malik & Coulson, 2008). Communication technologies offer a variety of opportunities for patients to acquire and share health-related information.

Acquiring and sharing health information can have a variety potential benefits and limitations for patients. Health information can serve to help manage uncertainty (Brashers, 2001) as well as increase patients' knowledge and engagement in their care (Lambert & Loiselle, 2007). There are, however, potential drawbacks to acquiring and sharing health information. Health information can make it difficult to manage uncertainty if it is contradictory or the volume is overwhelming (Brashers, Goldsmith, & Hsieh,

2002). Additionally, patients may experience anxiety when they are not able to obtain the information they desire (Lambert & Loiselle, 2007).

Reinforcing and Expanding Social Connections   A fourth form of coping involves bolstering existing connections and expanding one's social network. Communication technologies can be used to strengthen existing relationships with friends, family, and health providers. Mothers in one study who blogged more frequently reported greater feelings of connection with existing friends and family member (McDaniel, Coyne, & Holmes, 2012). E-mail was perceived to be a means for health providers to develop stronger relationships with their patients (Moyer, Stern, Dobias, Cox, & Katz, 2002). Communication technologies were also key in expanding patients' social networks. Online support communities provided a means to connect with previously unknown others who were experiencing similar health issues (Haberstroh & Moyer, 2012; Høybye, Johansen, & Tjørnhøj-Thomsen, 2005). A sense of inclusion or decreased isolation from forming new connections online was evident among bloggers writing about obesity (Dickins, Browning, Feldman, & Thomas, 2016) and in the comments left on a video-sharing website in response to videos of people describing their experiences with serious mental illness (Naslund, Grande, Aschbrenner, & Elwyn, 2014). In these ways, communication technologies can create opportunities for patients to strengthen their existing relationships and grow their social network.

Reinforcing and expanding social connections can be beneficial to patients as means to acquire social support. Patients can gain access to information, comfort, or other resources by virtue of their social relationships (MacGeorge, Feng, & Burleson, 2011). Some drawbacks of social relationships also exist. One's connections may intentionally or unintentionally behave in unhelpful ways or otherwise make coping more difficult (Dakof & Taylor, 1990; Figueiredo, Fries, & Ingram, 2004).

Creating a Legacy   A final coping activity germane to communication technology use among patients is defining one's legacy. Creating a legacy involves attempting to leave something behind for others from one's life or illness experience. Health bloggers were motivated to leave a record of their lives for their children (Chiu & Hsieh, 2013). Online community members shared their illness experiences in hopes that others dealing with similar circumstances would learn from them (Attard & Coulson, 2012). Family members and friends of people who committed suicide participated in online memorials for the deceased to help defend the deceased's actions and account for their death (Leonard & Toller, 2012). Communication technologies make it possible to construct and manage one's legacy.

Creating a legacy can be important to patients and their loved ones. It can help patients maintain a sense of dignity as they approach death (Hunter, 2008). Intervention studies have shown that legacy building can also promote better relationships between terminal patients and their families and leave a lasting record for future generations (Allen, Hilgeman, Ege, Shuster, & Burgio, 2008; Bernat, Helft, Wilhelm, Schmidt, & Johns, 2014). Yet it also seems possible that creating a legacy may cause distress as patients contemplate the end of life. Additionally, reading or viewing a deceased patient's online legacy may create challenges for family members or friends in recovering from their loss.

Situational and Individual Difference Factors

In addition to the three primary components of the digital coping model, a final set of factors are included to account for situational and individual differences in the salience of particular communication technology affordances. Patients' personality, social environment, and health condition may all influence their perceptions and use of specific affordances for digital coping. Several more specific variables are identified within each of these three categories. It should be noted that the individual variables discussed in the following paragraphs are intended to be representative and not exhaustive. It is possible that additional variables may exist within each category that could be systematically related to affordance perceptions.

Intrapersonal Predictors Several intrapersonal factors may serve to make particular communication technologies more or less salient to patients engaged in digital coping. These factors are dispositional in that they are stable personality-like characteristics that originate within patients. Four traits that may be important include extraversion, conscientiousness, tolerance for uncertainty, and optimism.

Extraversion is a personality trait that involves being outgoing, assertive, and active (John, Naumann, & Soto, 2008). It has been linked with better health and perceptions of health behavior (Williams, O'Brien, & Colder,

2004). Patients who are more extraverted may be drawn to the visibility affordance of communication technologies. Because they are sociable, extraverted patients may be particularly inclined to make themselves visible to others or to observe others' behavior. *Conscientiousness* is a second personality trait that concerns beings being disciplined, organized, and forward-thinking (John et al., 2008). Conscientiousness has been found to be correlated with better physical and mental health (Goodwin & Friedman, 2006). The documentation affordance of communication technologies may be particularly salient to patients who are more conscientious. The potential to make and keep a record would be valuable for organization and making plans.

Intolerance for uncertainty involves a negative reaction to situations marked by uncertainty (Freeston, Rhéaume, Letarte, Dugas, & Ladouceur, 1994) and has been connected with health monitoring in prior research (Rosen, Knäuper, & Sammut, 2007). The diversity affordance may be especially salient to patients with a greater intolerance for uncertainty. The potential to access diverse sources and information would make it possible for patients to potentially reduce or prospectively prevent uncertainty related to their illness. *Optimism* reflects a general tendency to expect positive rather than negative outcomes and has been associated with active coping efforts and better physical health (Carver, Scheier, & Segerstrom, 2010). Optimistic patients may be drawn to the visibility affordance of communication technologies. Their positive outcome expectations may lead them to see the potential benefits of sharing their experiences by making them visible to others.

Social Predictors Beyond intrapersonal characteristics, several interpersonal or social factors may lead communication technology affordances to be salient among patients. Social factors involve or are influenced by the social environment in which patients are situated. Stigma, communication efficacy, support availability, and social anxiety are four specific factors relevant to patients.

Stigma has traditionally been defined as a mark of discredit recognized by a social group (Goffman, 1963). In the context of health, stigma involves the perception that one's health condition is discrediting and can lead to social rejection or otherwise cause patients to withdraw from social groups to avoid harm (R. A. Smith, 2007). By virtue of making patients wary of experiencing retribution for their health condition, stigma could make the anonymity affordance of communication technologies salient. Concealing their identity could offer a means of protection for patients who feel stigmatized. *Communication efficacy* involves a patient's belief that he or she has the ability to successfully complete a communication activity (Afifi & Weiner, 2004). It has been linked with the propensity to perform behaviors such as health information seeking (Afifi & Weiner, 2006). Patients who lack communication efficacy may be particularly drawn to the control affordance. The potential for interactional control may be viewed as a way to counter difficulties expressing ideas or requesting information.

Social support availability refers to patients' general perceptions that, if called on, they have people who they can count on for assistance (Helgeson, 1993). Among patients, greater perceptions of support availability could make the reach affordance salient. Patients who recognize the presence of potential help providers may be inclined to use communication technologies to seek out these specific individuals. *Social anxiety* involves concerns with being evaluated or scrutinized by others (Segrin, 2001). People who are socially anxious have difficulty forming and maintaining relationships. Given their concern with social evaluation, the control affordance could be salient among patients with social anxiety. The potential to manage aspects of interaction may help patients with social anxiety feel more comfortable communicating with others.

Illness-Related Predictors Finally, factors related to the health condition experienced by patients may make some affordances salient. Four that are likely to be important involve the duration, intensity, history, and prognosis of the condition. As with the other factors, these four predictors are intended to be representative and not comprehensive. It is certainly possible that other illness-related factors may influence patients' perceptions of communication technology affordances.

Duration involves whether the illness is chronic or acute. When a condition is chronic, patients may be drawn to the documentation affordance of technologies to record and monitor their progress or experiences. *Intensity* refers to the level of immediate burden placed on patients by a health condition. Burden can involve the level of impairment, time obligation, or several other dimensions. The key factor in intensity is that illness places substantial and pressing demands on patients. When intensity increases, the availability affordance should become salient as patients seek to meet their immediate needs.

History involves the degree to which a specific illness-related issue is new or continuing. For any specific health condition, several unique symptoms, problems, or concerns may arise. The affordance of diversity may be salient when facing new issues. Diverse types of information may be particularly desirable to help understand and respond to novel issues. *Prognosis* concerns the potential outcomes of a health condition. When patients perceive death as a legitimate possibility, the documentation affordance may be particularly salient. Patients may be motivated to leave a formal record of their existence.

Functions of the Digital Coping Model

Having considered the key elements of the digital coping model, it is important to explain the model's functions. As previously discussed, a central objective in developing the model is to bring order to the diverse body of research focused on the use and implications of communication technologies among patients. To that end, the model helps to describe the core components involved in digital coping. Three basic elements have been identified: forms of distress, affordances of communication technologies, and coping activities. The forms of distress are akin to primary appraisals and involve disturbances commonly observed among people engaging in digital coping. The technological affordances function in secondary appraisals. They are assessments of the opportunities provided by technologies for action in responding to illness-related stressors. Three categories of factors that can influence the salience of affordances also have been identified. The digital coping activities are particular lines of behavior enacted using communication technologies in responding to a stressor. They involve efforts to ameliorate or manage a specific form of distress. Taken together, these three elements—sources of distress, technological affordances, and coping activities—serve to explain what is involved in digital coping.

Beyond identifying the major elements, a second function of the model is to detail the broader process of digital coping. Although the model is primarily intended to be descriptive, it is possible to make some predictions about when and how patients may use communication technologies to engage in digital coping. One general prediction involves the connection between appraisals and digital coping efforts. Lazarus and colleagues

(Lazarus, 1966, 2012; Lazarus & Folkman, 1984) noted that coping involves a process of responding to a stressor. In their work, primary and secondary appraisals functioned together and served to influence coping activities aimed at addressing the stressor. In the digital coping model, forms of distress and perceptions of affordances similarly represent an appraisal of the situation, along with opportunities presented by communication technologies. Together they are predicted to shape coping activities. That is, digital coping activities stem from the nature of distress experienced by patients and their perceptions of communication technology affordances. In considering this prediction, it is important to keep in mind that many situations will involve more than one form of distress, and several affordances may be relevant.

The digital coping model is distinct from other theoretical frameworks involving coping in that communication technologies play a central role. Accordingly, three sets of more focused predictions are possible that directly address the use and functions of affordances. To reiterate, any combination of distress and affordance could lead to each of the digital coping activities. It seems likely, however, that some general trends exist in the connections between affordance perceptions/use and distress, individual differences/ situational factors, and digital coping activities.

First, the forms of distress identified during primary appraisals may be systematically connected with the affordances targeted during secondary appraisals. In Lazarus and colleagues' (Lazarus, 1966, 2012; Lazarus & Folkman, 1984) work on stress and coping, primary and secondary appraisals occur in sequence. An assessment of what is happening is followed by an evaluation of one's resources for responding. As such, the stressor one is experiencing could influence the response options one considers. In the digital coping model, the forms of distress represent common stressors faced by patients. These forms of distress similarly may influence the types of affordances patients consider. Although any single affordance could possibly be used in response to each of the forms of distress, it seems likely that some trends in the nature of distress and specific affordance are used by digital patients.

Patients experiencing emotional upset should be especially likely to make use of the availability and anonymity affordances. Availability makes it possible for people experiencing upset to immediately deal with their distress. Anonymity can be important for addressing any embarrassment or social discomfort associated with aversive emotions. When inadequate information is a source of distress, it should be connected with patients' use of the control, diversity, and reach affordances. Control makes it possible for patients to regulate their efforts to acquire or avoid information, whereas diversity offers the opportunity to connect with different types of information sources. Reach makes it possible to locate a specific piece of information or information source.

Distress stemming from insufficient support should lead patients to use the visibility affordance in an effort to identify and expose themselves to others and the reach affordance to locate specific support providers. Patients experiencing physical pain should be likely to use the availability affordance to quickly deal with their discomfort. Finally, distress resulting from existential concerns should be connected to use of the documentation affordance. Documentation offers a potential for permanence that could be valuable in confronting existential issues. Each of these specific predictions is summarized in table 8.1. It is important to reiterate that they represent general trends expected in the nature of affordances identified during secondary appraisals stemming from the form of distress experienced by patients. It is possible for individual patients to use virtually any of the affordances in response to the various forms of distress.

A second set of predictions can be made regarding those personality and situational variables that might lead particular affordances of communication technologies to be more or less salient. As previously discussed, patients' personality, social environment, and health condition are three general classes of factors that can contribute to affordance salience. These factors can lead patients to recognize the affordance, perceive its utility, and/or employ it in digital coping. Patients, for example, who are more extraverted may be drawn to the visibility affordance because it facilitates sociability by allowing them to be seen and observe others. The anonymity affordance may be particularly salient to patients who perceive their illness to be stigmatized and wish to reduce the potential of (offline) discrimination. Although a comprehensive list of individual factors within each of the three categories is beyond the scope of this project, a number of exemplars were outlined previously in this chapter. The specific predictions stemming from those exemplars are summarized in table 8.2.

A third set of predictions involves trends in the types of coping activities for which affordances are used. Affordances are more or less likely to

Table 8.1
Trends in Affordances Selected by Patients Based on Forms of Distress

Forms of Distress	Affordances						
	Anonymity	Availability	Control	Diversity	Documentation	Reach	Visibility
Emotional upset	+						
Inadequate information		+	+	+		+	
Insufficient support						+	+
Physical pain		+					
Existential concerns					+		

+ Indicates that an affordance is likely to be connected with a form of distress.

Table 8.2
Trends in Affordance Perceptions/Use Based on Personality/Situational Factors

	Affordances						
	Anonymity	Availability	Control	Diversity	Documentation	Reach	Visibility
Intrapersonal factors							
Extraversion							+
Conscientiousness					+		
Uncertainty intolerance				+			
Optimism							+
Social factors							
Stigma	+						
Comm. efficacy			+				
Support availability						+	
Social anxiety			+				
Illness-related factors							
Duration					+		
Intensity		+					
History				+			
Prognosis					+		

+ Indicates that a specific factor is likely to be connected with perceptions/use of an affordance.

facilitate particular coping behaviors. When a given affordance is salient, patients may be especially likely to engage in certain coping activities. Specific predictions are summarized in table 8.3 and discussed in the following paragraphs.

When the anonymity affordance is salient, patients should be especially likely to engage in sense-making, managing upset, and acquiring/sharing information. Each of these coping activities can involve revealing information that could be embarrassing or otherwise threaten one's image or reputation. Through making it possible for patients to conceal their identity, anonymity could mitigate such concerns and make it easier to perform these three coping activities. Trends also should exist in the coping activities enacted when the availability affordance is salient. This affordance should be particularly useful in facilitating coping activities that involve responding to a pressing problem or threat, such as managing upset, acquiring/sharing information, and reinforcing/expanding connections.

When the diversity affordance is salient, patients should be likely to engage in managing upset or acquiring/sharing information. The ability to gain access to multiple perspectives should provide opportunities for responding to upset and finding information. The documentation affordance should encourage coping activities that would benefit from having or being able to retain a formal written record such as sense-making, acquiring/sharing information, and creating a legacy. The visibility affordance makes it possible to observe others behavior or have one's behavior observed. It would be especially useful in activities where access to others would be beneficial such as acquiring/sharing information, reinforce/expand connections, or creating a legacy.

When the reach affordance is salient, patients should be likely to engage in managing upset, acquiring/sharing information, and reinforcing/expanding connections. Each of these three activities could be facilitated by the potential to access specific people or information. Finally, any of the five coping activities may follow when the control affordance is salient to patients. The potential to manage aspects of interaction would be equally valuable for performing each coping activity. In considering these predictions, it should be noted that they do not extend to the effectiveness of coping efforts. Although an affordance may facilitate a given coping activity, that activity may not necessarily lead to objectively beneficial coping outcomes.

Table 8.3
Trends in Digital Coping Activities Based on Affordance Use

Affordances	Digital Coping Activities				
	Sense-Making	Managing Upset	Acquiring/Sharing Information	Reinforcing/Expanding Connections	Creating a Legacy
Anonymity	+				+
Availability		+	+	+	
Control	+	+	+		
Documentation	+		+		
Diversity		+	+		
Reach			+	+	
Visibility		+	+	+	+

+ Indicates that an affordance is likely to be connected with a digital coping activity.

Implications of the Digital Coping Model

The digital coping model has potential utility for both health care professionals and researchers. The model privileges the role of communication technologies in the coping process by focusing on the opportunities they can provide for responding to distress. It offers a framework for identifying how and why communication technologies are perceived and used by patients.

For health care professionals, the model offers insights about what it means to be a patient in the digital age. Communication technologies are a pervasive part of contemporary life—and, as evidenced throughout this book, their use extends to coping with illness. Understanding how and why these technologies are used by the lay public can be of great value to health care professionals. The forms of distress considered in the model represent the major classes of stressors experienced by digital patients. The affordances similarly highlight those aspects of communication technologies that are particularly salient to patients and may be leveraged to facilitate coping efforts. The coping strategies offer further insights about the specific ways that these technologies are used to respond to stressors as well as some potential benefits and limitations of these activities.

In better understanding how these technologies are perceived and used, health care professionals will be able to more effectively advise and manage patients engaging in digital coping efforts. Health care professionals can see communication technologies from a patient's perspective and, as a result, respond to patients more effectively. Understanding, for example, the various types of affordances will allow health care professionals to recognize their potential and pitfalls and advise patients accordingly. Similarly, knowing the different digital coping strategies will position health care professionals to appreciate what patients are attempting to accomplish in using communication technologies and how those objectives might be achieved.

For researchers, the model advances our understanding of how technologies are used among people experiencing illness. It elucidates the connections between dimensions of illness (i.e., source of distress), perceptions of technologies (i.e., affordances), and specific uses of technologies for coping. More generally, the model helps to organize and synthesize a disconnected body of research. Research on digital coping can be found in an impressive range of fields from the social sciences to computer science and medicine. The model serves to identify and describe those pervasive elements of digital coping. It is noteworthy that these elements transcend individual technologies and health conditions. As such, the model offers a broad and potentially robust framework for explaining digital coping.

The digital coping model can also guide and spur future scholarship. At the most basic level, it offers a framework for examining the role of communication technologies in coping with illness. In identifying the key components of digital coping, the model helps focus researchers on those factors that are likely to be most consequential. Moreover, the model underscores the importance of examining factors that transcend individual technologies and illnesses. It is not being argued that studies of individual technologies or illnesses lack value. Rather, through studying universal elements of technologies and illness, researchers are likely to make the greatest contributions to the understanding of digital coping.

Conclusion

As communication technologies become increasingly integrated into the everyday lives of people around the world, it seems reasonable to expect their implications for patients to grow. The central objective of this book has been to synthesize the diverse body of research on this phenomenon and advance an original model of digital coping. Grounded in established theory about stress and coping, the model serves to explain why and how communication technologies are used in coping with illness. The perceived affordances of communication technologies are proposed to combine with the nature of the stressor experienced by patients to encourage specific coping activities. The digital coping model offers researchers and health care professionals a general guide to understand the uses and effects of communication technologies among patients. Through the continued efforts of both groups, it is my sincere hope that we can minimize the burden of illness and better the lives of patients.

References

Abrahamson, J. A., Fisher, K. E., Turner, A. G., Durrance, J. C., & Turner, T. C. (2008). Lay information mediary behavior uncovered: Exploring how nonprofessionals seek health information for themselves and others online. *Journal of the Medical Library Association: JMLA, 96*(4), 310–323. doi:10.3163/1536-5050.96.4.006.

Afifi, W. A., & Weiner, J. L. (2004). Toward a theory of motivated information management. *Communication Theory, 14*(2), 167–190. doi:10.1111/j.1468-2885.2004.tb00310.x.

Afifi, W. A., & Weiner, J. L. (2006). Seeking information about sexual health: Applying the theory of motivated information management. *Human Communication Research, 32*(1), 35–57. doi:10.1111/j.1468-2958.2006.00002.x.

Ahluwalia, S., Murray, E., Stevenson, F., Kerr, C., & Burns, J. (2010). "A heartbeat moment": Qualitative study of GP views of patients bringing health information from the internet to a consultation. *British Journal of General Practice, 60*(571), 88–94. doi:10.3399/bjgp10X483120.

Allen, R. S., Hilgeman, M. M., Ege, M. A., Shuster, J. L., & Burgio, L. D. (2008). Legacy activities as interventions approaching the end of life. *Journal of Palliative Medicine, 11*(7), 1029–1038. doi:10.1089/jpm.2007.0294.

Almalki, M., Gray, K., & Martin-Sanchez, F. (2016). Activity theory as a theoretical framework for health self-quantification: A systematic review of empirical studies. *Journal of Medical Internet Research, 18*(5), e131. doi:10.2196/jmir.5000.

Anand, S. G., Feldman, M. J., Geller, D. S., Bisbee, A., & Bauchner, H. (2005). A content analysis of e-mail communication between primary care providers and parents. *Pediatrics, 115*(5), 1283–1288. doi:10.1542/peds.2004-1297.

Andersen, T., & Ruland, C. M. (2009). Cancer patients' questions and concerns expressed in an online nurse-delivered mail service: Preliminary results. *Studies in Health Technology and Informatics, 146*, 149–153.

Andreassen, H. K., Trondsen, M., Kummervold, P. E., Gammon, D., & Hjortdahl, P. (2006). Patients who use e-mediated communication with their doctor: New constructions of trust in the patient-doctor relationship. *Qualitative Health Research*, *16*(2), 238–248. doi:10.1177/1049732305284667.

Anonymous. (1998). To reveal or not to reveal: A theoretical model of anonymous communication. *Communication Theory*, *8*(4), 381-407. doi:10.1111/j.1468-2885.1998. tb00226.x.

Antheunis, M. L., Tates, K., & Nieboer, T. E. (2013). Patients' and health professionals' use of social media in health care: Motives, barriers and expectations. *Patient Education and Counseling*, *92*(3), 426–431. doi:10.1016/j.pec.2013.06.020.

Arntson, P., & Droge, D. (1987). Social support in self-help groups: The role of communication in enabling perceptions of control. In T. L. Albrecht & M. B. Adelman (Eds.), *Communicating social support* (pp. 148–171). Newbury Park, CA: Sage.

Askelson, N. M., Campo, S., & Carter, K. D. (2011). Completely isolated? Health information seeking among social isolates. *Health Education & Behavior*, *38*(2), 116–122.

Attard, A., & Coulson, N. S. (2012). A thematic analysis of patient communication in Parkinson's disease online support group discussion forums. *Computers in Human Behavior*, *28*(2), 500–506. doi:10.1016/j.chb.2011.10.022.

Aung, K.-K., Wu, W. K., Tokumi, A., Kuo, P., & Day, C. S. (2015). Does a directive to an Internet site enhance the doctor-patient interaction? A prospective randomized study for patients with carpal tunnel syndrome. *Journal of Bone and Joint Surgery*, *97*(13), 1112–1118. doi:10.2106/JBJS.N.00741.

Balka, E., Krueger, G., Holmes, B. J., & Stephen, J. E. (2010). Situating internet use: Information-seeking among young women with breast cancer. *Journal of Computer-Mediated Communication*, *15*(3), 389–411. doi:10.1111/j.1083-6101.2010.01506.x.

Bar-Lev, S. (2008). "We are here to give you emotional support": Performing emotions in an online HIV/AIDS support group. *Qualitative Health Research*, *18*(4), 509–521. doi:10.1177/1049732307311680.

Bashshur, R. L., & Shannon, G. W. (2009). *History of telemedicine*. New Rochelle, NY: Mary Ann Liebert.

Baur, C. (2000). Limiting factors on the transformative powers of e-mail in patient-physician relationships: A critical analysis. *Health Communication*, *12*(3), 239–259.

Bazarova, N. N., & Choi, Y. H. (2014). Self-disclosure in social media: Extending the functional approach to disclosure motivations and characteristics on social network sites. *Journal of Communication*, *64*(4), 635–657. doi:10.1111/jcom.12106.

Beaudoin, C. E., & Hong, T. (2011). Health information seeking, diet and physical activity: An empirical assessment by medium and critical demographics. *International Journal of Medical Informatics, 80*(8), 586–595. doi:10.1016/j.ijmedinf.2011.04.003.

Beckjord, E. B., Finney Rutten, L. J., Volckmann, L., Hesse, B. W., Squiers, L., Arora, N. K., & Hesse, B. W. (2007). Use of the Internet to communicate with health care providers in the United States: Estimates from the 2003 and 2005 Health Information National Trends Surveys (HINTS). *Journal of Medical Internet Research, 9*(3). doi:10.2196/jmir.9.3.e20.

Bell, R. A., Hu, X., Orrange, S. E., & Kravitz, R. L. (2011). Lingering questions and doubts: Online information-seeking of support forum members following their medical visits. *Patient Education and Counseling, 85*(3), 525–528. doi:10.1016/j.pec.2011.01.015.

Berger, M., Wagner, T. H., & Baker, L. C. (2005). Internet use and stigmatized illness. *Social Science & Medicine, 61*(8), 1821–1827. doi:10.1016/j.socscimed.2005.03.025.

Berkman, L. F., & Glass, T. (2000). Social integration, social networks, social support, and health. *Social Epidemiology, 1*, 137–173. doi:10.1016/S0277-9536(00)00065-4.

Bernat, J. K., Helft, P. R., Wilhelm, L. R., Schmidt, K., & Johns, S. A. (2014). Creating communicative opportunity: The supportive benefits of legacy building for families of advanced cancer patients. *Journal of Clinical Oncology, 32*, 230. doi:10.1200/jco.2014.32.31_suppl.230.

Bhandari, N., Shi, Y., & Jung, K. (2014). Seeking health information online: Does limited healthcare access matter? *Journal of the American Medical Informatics Association, 21*(6), 1113–1117. doi:10.1136/amiajnl-2013-002350.

Blight, M. G., Jagiello, K., & Ruppel, E. K. (2015). "Same stuff different day:" A mixed-method study of support seeking on Facebook. *Computers in Human Behavior, 53*, 366–373. doi:10.1016/j.chb.2015.07.029.

Bodie, G. D., & Burleson, B. R. (2008). Explaining variations in the effects of supportive messages: A dual-process framework. In C. Beck (Ed.), *Communication yearbook* (Vol. 32, pp. 355–398). New York: Routledge.

Bolger, N., Zuckerman, A., & Kessler, R. C. (2000). Invisible support and adjustment to stress. *Journal of Personality and Social Psychology, 79*(6), 953–961. doi:10.1037/0022-3514.79.6.953.

Boniel-Nissim, M., & Barak, A. (2013). The therapeutic value of adolescents' blogging about social—emotional difficulties. *Psychological Services, 10*(3), 333–341. doi:10.1037/a0026664.

Boot, C. R. L., & Meijman, F. J. (2010). The public and the Internet: Multifaceted drives for seeking health information. *Health Informatics Journal, 16*(2), 145–156. doi:10.1177/1460458210364786.

Bosslet, G. T., Torke, A. M., Hickman, S. E., Terry, C. L., & Helft, P. R. (2011). The patient—doctor relationship and online social networks: Results of a national survey. *Journal of General Internal Medicine, 26*(10), 1168–1174. doi:10.1007/s11606-011-1761-2.

Bowes, P., Stevenson, F., Ahluwalia, S., & Murray, E. (2012). "I need her to be a doctor": Patients' experiences of presenting health information from the internet in GP consultations. *British Journal of General Practice, 62*(604), e732–e738. doi:10.3399/bjgp12X658250.

Brashers, D. E. (2001). Communication and uncertainty management. *Journal of Communication, 51*(3), 477–497. doi:10.1111/j.1460-2466.2001.tb02892.x.

Brashers, D. E., Goldsmith, D. J., & Hsieh, E. (2002). Information seeking and avoiding in health contexts. *Human Communication Research, 28*(2), 258–271. doi:10.1111/j.1468-2958.2002.tb00807.x.

Brigo, F., & Trinka, E. (2015). Google search behavior for status epilepticus. *Epilepsy & Behavior, 49*, 146–149. doi:10.1016/j.yebeh.2015.02.029.

Brissette, I., Cohen, S., & Seeman, T. E. (2000). *Measuring social integration and social networks*. New York: Oxford University Press.

Brooks, R. G., & Menachemi, N. (2006). Physicians' use of email with patients: Factors influencing electronic communication and adherence to best practices. *Journal of Medical Internet Research, 8*(1), 15–24. doi:10.2196/jmir.8.1.e2.

Broom, A. (2005a). Medical specialists' accounts of the impact of the Internet on the doctor/patient relationship. *Health, 9*(3), 319–338. doi:10.1177/1363459305052903.

Broom, A. (2005b). Virtually healthy: The impact of Internet use on disease experience and the doctor-patient relationship. *Qualitative Health Research, 15*(3), 325–345. doi:10.1177/1049732304272916.

Brown, J., Ryan, C., & Harris, A. (2014). How doctors view and use social media: A national survey. *Journal of Medical Internet Research, 16*(12), e267. doi:10.2196/jmir.3589.

Brown, J. B., Stewart, M., & Ryan, B. L. (2003). Outcomes of patient-provider interaction. In T. L. Thompson, A. M. Dorsey, K. I. Miller, & R. Parrott (Eds.), *Handbook of health communication* (pp. 141–163). Mahwah, NJ: Lawrence Erlbaum Associates.

Brubaker, J. R., Hayes, G. R., & Dourish, P. (2013). Beyond the grave: Facebook as a site for the expansion of death and mourning. *Information Society, 29*(3), 152–163. doi:10.1080/01972243.2013.777300.

Brusilovskiy, E., Townley, G., Snethen, G., & Salzer, M. S. (2016). Social media use, community participation and psychological well-being among individuals with serious mental illnesses. *Computers in Human Behavior, 65,* 232–240. doi:10.1016/j. chb.2016.08.036.

Buis, L. R. (2008). Emotional and informational support messages in an online hospice support community. *Computers, Informatics, Nursing. CIN, 26*(6), 358–367. doi:10.1097/01.NCN.0000336461.94939.97.

Bulled, N. (2011). "You can find anything online": Biocommunicability of cyber-health information and its impact on how the NET Generation accesses health care. *Human Organization, 70*(2), 153–163.

Bunde, M., Suls, J., Martin, R., & Barnett, K. (2006). Hystersisters online: Social support and social comparison among hysterectomy patients on the Internet. *Annals of Behavioral Medicine, 31*(3), 271–278. doi:10.1207/s15324796abm3103_9.

Burke, M., Kraut, R., & Williams, D. (2010). Social use of computer-mediated communication by adults on the autism spectrum. In *Proceedings of the 2010 ACM Conference on Computer Supported Cooperative Work* (pp. 425–434). New York, NY: ACM. doi:10.1145/1718918.1718991.

Burleson, B. R. (1994). Comforting messages: Features, functions, and outcomes. In J. A. Daly & J. M. Wiemann (Eds.), *Strategic interpersonal communication* (pp. 135–161). Hillsdale, NJ: Lawrence Erlbaum Associates.

Burleson, B. R., & Goldsmith, D. J. (1998). How the comforting process works: Alleviating emotional distress through conversationally induced reappraisals. In P. A. Andersen & L. K. Guerrero (Eds.), *Handbook of communication and emotion: Research, theory, applications, and contexts* (pp. 245–280). San Diego, CA: Academic Press.

Bury, M. (1982). Chronic illness as biographical disruption. *Sociology of Health & Illness, 4*(2), 167–182. doi:10.1111/1467-9566.ep11339939.

Bylund, C. L. (2005). Mothers' involvement in decision making during the birthing process: A quantitative analysis of women's online birth stories. *Health Communication, 18*(1), 23–39. doi:10.1207/s15327027hc1801_2.

Bylund, C. L., Gueguen, J. A., D'Agostino, T. A., Li, Y., & Sonet, E. (2010). Doctor—patient communication about cancer-related internet information. *Journal of Psychosocial Oncology, 28*(2), 127–142. doi:10.1080/07347330903570495.

Caiata-Zufferey, M., & Schulz, P. J. (2012). Physicians' communicative strategies in interacting with Internet-informed patients: Results from a qualitative study. *Health Communication, 27*(8), 738–749. doi:10.1080/10410236.2011.636478.

Capitulo, K. L. (2004). Perinatal grief online. *The American Journal of Maternal/Child Nursing, 29*(5), 305–311. doi:10.1097/00005721-200409000-00008.

Caplan, S. E., & Turner, J. S. (2007). Bringing theory to research on computer-mediated supportive and comforting communication. *Computers in Human Behavior, 23*, 985–998. doi:10.1016/j.chb.2005.08.003.

Carpenter, C. J., & Amaravadi, C. S. (2016). A big data approach to assessing the impact of social norms: Reporting one's exercise to a social media audience. *Communication Research* [Advanced online publication]. doi:10.1177/0093650216657776.

Carroll, B., & Landry, K. (2010). Logging on and letting out: Using online social networks to grieve and to mourn. *Bulletin of Science, Technology & Society, 30*(5), 341–349. doi:10.1177/0270467610380006.

Carron-Arthur, B., Ali, K., Cunningham, A. J., & Griffiths, M. K. (2015). From help-seekers to influential users: A systematic review of participation styles in online health communities. *Journal of Medical Internet Research, 17*(12), e271. doi:10.2196/jmir.4705.

Carron-Arthur, B., Reynolds, J., Bennett, K., Bennett, A., Cunningham, J. A., & Griffiths, K. M. (2016). Community structure of a mental health Internet support group: Modularity in user thread participation. *JMIR Mental Health, 3*(2), e20. doi:10.2196/mental.4961.

Carver, C. S., Scheier, M. F., & Segerstrom, S. C. (2010). Optimism. *Clinical Psychology Review, 30*(7), 879–889. doi:10.1016/j.cpr.2010.01.006.

Carver, C. S., Scheier, M. F., & Weintraub, J. K. (1989). Assessing coping strategies: A theoretically based approach. *Journal of Personality and Social Psychology, 56*(2), 267–283. doi:10.1037/0022-3514.56.2.267.

Case, D. O. (2007). *Looking for information.* London, UK: Elsevier.

Centola, D. (2010). The spread of behavior in an online social network experiment. *Science, 329*(5996), 1194–1197. doi:10.1126/science.1185231.

Centola, D. (2011). An experimental study of homophily in the adoption of health behavior. *Science, 334*(6060), 1269–1272. doi:10.1126/science.1207055.

Centola, D., & Macy, M. (2007). Complex contagions and the weakness of long ties. *American Journal of Sociology, 113*(3), 702–734. doi:10.1086/521848.

Centola, D., & van de Rijt, A. (2015). Choosing your network: Social preferences in an online health community. *Social Science & Medicine, 125*, 19–31. doi:10.1016/j.socscimed.2014.05.019.

Chae, J. (2015). Online cancer information seeking increases cancer worry. *Computers in Human Behavior, 52*, 144–150. doi:10.1016/j.chb.2015.05.019.

Chang, H.-J. (2009). Online supportive interactions: Using a network approach to examine communication patterns within a psychosis social support group in

Taiwan. *Journal of the American Society for Information Science and Technology*, *60*(7), 1504–1517. doi:10.1002/asi.21070.

Chang, P. F., & Bazarova, N. N. (2016). Managing stigma: Disclosure-response communication patterns in pro-anorexic websites. *Health Communication*, *31*(2), 217–229. doi:10.1080/10410236.2014.946218.

Chapple, A., & Ziebland, S. (2011). How the Internet is changing the experience of bereavement by suicide: A qualitative study in the UK. *Health*, *15*(2), 173–187. doi:10.1177/1363459309360792.

Charles, C., Gafni, A., & Whelan, T. (1997). Shared decision-making in the medical encounter: What does it mean? (Or it takes at least two to tango). *Social Science & Medicine*, *44*(5), 681–692. doi:10.1016/S0277-9536(96)00221-3.

Chen, A. T. (2012a). Exploring online support spaces: Using cluster analysis to examine breast cancer, diabetes and fibromyalgia support groups. *Patient Education and Counseling*, *87*(2), 250–257. doi:10.1016/j.pec.2011.08.017.

Chen, A. T. (2012b). Information seeking over the course of illness: The experience of people with fibromyalgia. *Musculoskeletal Care*, *10*(4), 212–220. doi:10.1002/msc.1022.

Chisolm, D. J. (2010). Does online health information seeking act like a health behavior? A test of the behavioral model. *Telemedicine Journal and e-Health*, *16*(2), 154–160. doi:10.1089/tmj.2009.0102.

Chiu, Y.-C. (2011). Probing, impelling, but not offending doctors: The role of the internet as an information source for patients' interactions with doctors. *Qualitative Health Research*, *21*(12), 1658–1666. doi:10.1177/1049732311417455.

Chiu, Y.-C., & Hsieh, Y.-L. (2013). Communication online with fellow cancer patients: Writing to be remembered, gain strength, and find survivors. *Journal of Health Psychology*, *18*(12), 1572–1581. doi:10.1177/1359105312465915.

Choe, E. K., Lee, N. B., Lee, B., Pratt, W., & Kientz, J. A. (2014). Understanding quantified-selfers' practices in collecting and exploring personal data. In *Proceedings of the 32nd Annual ACM Conference on Human Factors in Computing Systems* (pp. 1143–1152). New York, NY: ACM. doi:10.1145/2556288.2557372.

Choi, Y. H., & Bazarova, N. N. (2015). Self-disclosure characteristics and motivations in social media: Extending the functional model to multiple social network sites. *Human Communication Research*, *41*(4), 480–500. doi:10.1111/hcre.12053.

Chomutare, T., Årsand, E., Fernandez-Luque, L., Lauritzen, J., & Hartvigsen, G. (2013). Inferring community structure in healthcare forums: An empirical study. *Methods of Information in Medicine*, *52*(2), 160–167. doi:10.3414/ME12-02-0003.

Chou, W.-Y. S., Hunt, Y., Folkers, A., & Augustson, E. (2011). Cancer survivorship in the age of YouTube and social media: A narrative analysis. *Journal of Medical Internet Research, 13*(1), e7. doi:10.2196/jmir.1569.

Choudhury, M. D., Morris, M. R., & White, R. W. (2014). Seeking and sharing health information online: comparing search engines and social media. In *Proceedings of the SIGCHI Conference on Human Factors in Computing Systems* (pp. 1365–1376). New York, NY: ACM. doi:10.1145/2556288.2557214.

Chung, D. S., & Kim, S. (2008). Blogging activity among cancer patients and their companions: Uses, gratifications, and predictors of outcomes. *Journal of the American Society for Information Science and Technology, 59*(2), 297–306. doi:10.1002/asi.20751.

Chung, J. E. (2013). Social interaction in online support groups: Preference for online social interaction over offline social interaction. *Computers in Human Behavior, 29*(4), 1408–1414. doi:10.1016/j.chb.2013.01.019.

Chung, J. E. (2014). Social networking in online support groups for health: How online social networking benefits patients. *Journal of Health Communication, 19*(6), 639–659. doi:10.1080/10810730.2012.757396.

Church, S. H. (2013). Digital gravescapes: Digital memorializing on Facebook. *Information Society, 29*(3), 184–189. doi:10.1080/01972243.2013.777309.

Cobb, N. K., Graham, A. L., & Abrams, D. B. (2010). Social network structure of a large online community for smoking cessation. *American Journal of Public Health, 100*(7), 1282–1289. doi:10.2105/AJPH.2009.165449.

Cohen, G. E., & Kerr, B. A. (1999). Computer-mediated counseling: An empirical study of a new mental health treatment. *Computers in Human Services, 15*, 13–26. doi:10.1300/J407v15n04_02.

Cohen, S., Underwood, L., & Gottlieb, B. (2000). *Social support measurement and interventions: A guide for health and social scientists.* New York: Oxford.

Cohen, S., & Wills, T. A. (1985). Stress, social support and the buffering hypothesis. *Psychological Bulletin, 98*(2), 310–357. doi:10.1037/0033-2909.98.2.310.

Cole, J., Watkins, C., & Kleine, D. (2016). Health advice from Internet discussion forums: How bad is dangerous? *Journal of Medical Internet Research, 18*(1), e4. doi:10.2196/jmir.5051.

Colombo, C., Mosconi, P., Confalonieri, P., Baroni, I., Traversa, S., Hill, S. J., … Filippini, G. (2014). Web search behavior and information needs of people with multiple sclerosis: Focus group study and analysis of online postings. *Interactive Journal of Medical Research, 3*(3), e12. doi:10.2196/ijmr.3034.

Colvin, J., Chenoeth, L., Bold, M., & Harding, C. (2004). Caregivers of older adults: Advantages and disadvantages of Internet-based social support. *Family Relations, 53*, 49–57. doi:10.1111/j.1741-3729.2004.00008.x.

Cook, J. E., & Doyle, C. (2002). Working alliance in online therapy as compared to face-to-face therapy: Preliminary results. *Cyberpsychology & Behavior, 5*(2), 95–105. doi:10.1089/109493102753770480.

Cooper, C. P., Gelb, C. A., Rim, S. H., Hawkins, N. A., Rodriguez, J. L., & Polonec, L. (2012). Physicians who use social media and other internet-based communication technologies. *Journal of the American Medical Informatics Association, 19*(6), 960–964. doi:10.1136/amiajnl-2011-000628.

Cooper, C. P., Mallon, K. P., Leadbetter, S., Pollack, L. A., & Peipins, L. A. (2005). Cancer Internet search activity on a major search engine, United States 2001–2003. *Journal of Medical Internet Research, 7*(3), e36.

Cowles, K. V., & Rodgers, B. L. (1991). The concept of grief: A foundation for nursing research and practice. *Research in Nursing & Health, 14*(2), 119–127.

Crook, B., Glowacki, E. M., Love, B., Jones, B. L., Macpherson, C. F., & Johnson, R. H. (2015). Hanging by a thread: Exploring the features of nonresponse in an online young adult cancer survivorship support community. *Journal of Cancer Survivorship: Research and Practice, 10*(1), 185–193. doi:10.1007/s11764-015-0465-8.

Culnan, M. J., & Markus, M. L. (1987). Information technologies. In F. M. Jablin, L. L. Putnam, K. H. Roberts, & L. W. Porter (Eds.), *Handbook of organizational communication* (pp. 420–443). Newbury Park, CA: Sage.

Cummings, J. N., Sproull, L., & Kiesler, S. B. (2002). Beyond hearing: Where the real-world and online support meet. *Group Dynamics, 6*(1), 78–88. doi:10.1037/1089-2699.6.1.78.

Cutrona, C. E. (1990). Stress and social support: In search of optimal matching. *Journal of Social and Clinical Psychology, 9*, 3–14. doi:10.1521/jscp.1990.9.1.3.

Cutrona, C. E., & Russell, D. W. (1990). Type of social support and specific stress: Toward a theory of optimal matching. In B. R. Sarason, I. G. Sarason, & G. R. Pierce (Eds.), *Social support: An interactional view* (pp. 319–366). Oxford, England: John Wiley & Sons.

Cutrona, C. E., & Suhr, J. A. (1992). Controllability of stressful events and satisfaction with spouse support behaviors. *Communication Research, 19*(2), 154–174. doi:10.1177/009365092019002002.

Cutrona, S. L., Mazor, K. M., Vieux, S. N., Luger, T. M., Volkman, J. E., & Finney Rutten, L. J. (2015). Health information-seeking on behalf of others: Characteristics of "surrogate seekers." *Journal of Cancer Education, 30*(1), 12–19. doi:10.1007/s13187-014-0701-3.

D'Agostino, T. A., Ostroff, J. S., Heerdt, A., Dickler, M., Li, Y., & Bylund, C. L. (2012). Toward a greater understanding of breast cancer patients' decisions to discuss cancer-related internet information with their doctors: An exploratory study. *Patient Education and Counseling, 89*(1), 109–115. doi:10.1016/j.pec.2012.05.008.

Dakof, G. A., & Taylor, S. E. (1990). Victims' perceptions of social support: What is helpful from whom? *Journal of Personality and Social Psychology, 58*(1), 80–89. doi:10.1037/0022-3514.58.1.80.

Davison, K. P., Pennebaker, J. W., & Dickerson, S. S. (2000). Who talks? The social psychology of illness support groups. *American Psychologist, 55*(2), 205–217. doi:10.1037/0003-066X.55.2.205.

Day, M., Demiris, G., Oliver, D. P., Courtney, K., & Hensel, B. (2007). Exploring underutilization of videophones in hospice settings. *Telemedicine Journal and e-Health, 13*(1), 25–32. doi:10.1089/tmj.2006.0023.

De Rouck, S., & Leys, M. (2013). Illness trajectory and internet as a health information and communication channel used by parents of infants admitted to a neonatal intensive care unit. *Journal of Advanced Nursing, 69*(7), 1489–1499. doi:10.1111/jan.12007.

DeAndrea, D. C. (2015). Testing the proclaimed affordances of online support groups in a nationally representative sample of adults seeking mental health assistance. *Journal of Health Communication, 20*(2), 147–156. doi:10.1080/10810730.2014.914606.

DeAndrea, D. C., & Anthony, J. C. (2013). Online peer support for mental health problems in the United States: 2004–2010. *Psychological Medicine, 43*, 2277–2288. doi:10.1017/S0033291713000172.

DeGroot, J. M. (2012). Maintaining relational continuity with the deceased on Facebook. *Omega, 65*(3), 195–212. doi:10.2190/OM.65.3.c.

DeGroot, J. M. (2014). "For whom the bell tolls": Emotional rubbernecking in Facebook memorial groups. *Death Studies, 38*(2), 79–84. doi:10.1080/07481187.2012.725450.

Demiris, G., Oliver, D. P., Courtney, K. L., & Day, M. (2007). Telehospice tools for caregivers: A pilot study. *Clinical Gerontologist, 31*(1), 43–57. doi:10.1300/J018v31n01_04.

Demiris, G., Oliver, D. R. P., Fleming, D. A., & Edison, K. (2004). Hospice staff attitudes towards telehospice. *American Journal of Hospice & Palliative Medicine, 21*(5), 343–347. doi:10.1177/104990910402100507.

Demjén, Z. (2016). Laughing at cancer: Humour, empowerment, solidarity and coping online. *Journal of Pragmatics, 101*, 18–30. doi:10.1016/j.pragma.2016.05.010.

Derlega, V. J., Metts, S., Petronio, S., & Margulis, S. T. (1993). *Self-disclosure*. Thousand Oaks, CA: Sage.

Detz, A., López, A., & Sarkar, U. (2013). Long-term doctor-patient relationships: Patient perspective from online reviews. *Journal of Medical Internet Research, 15*(7), 112–121.

Dickins, M., Browning, C., Feldman, S., & Thomas, S. (2016). Social inclusion and the fatosphere: The role of an online weblogging community in fostering social inclusion. *Sociology of Health & Illness, 38,* 797–811. doi:10.1111/1467-9566. 12397.

Diviani, N., van den Putte, B., Giani, S., & van Weert, J. C. (2015). Low health literacy and evaluation of online health information: A systematic review of the literature. *Journal of Medical Internet Research, 17*(5), e112. doi:10.2196/jmir.4018.

Dobransky, K., & Hargittai, E. (2012). Inquiring minds acquiring wellness: Uses of online and offline sources for health information. *Health Communication, 27*(4), 331–343. doi:10.1080/10410236.2011.585451.

Dolce, M. C. (2011). The Internet as a source of health information: Experiences of cancer survivors and caregivers with healthcare providers. *Oncology Nursing Forum, 38*(3), 353–359. doi:10.1188/11.ONF.353-359.

Doolittle, G. C. (2000). A cost measurement study for a home-based telehospice service. *Journal of Telemedicine and Telecare, 6*(Suppl 1), S193–S195.

Doolittle, G. C., Yaezel, A., Otto, F., & Clemens, C. (1998). Hospice care using home-based telemedicine systems. *Journal of Telemedicine and Telecare, 4*(Suppl 1), 58–59. doi:10.1258/1357633981931470.

Döveling, K. (2015). Emotion regulation in bereavement: Searching for and finding emotional support in social network sites. *New Review of Hypermedia and Multimedia, 21*(1–2), 106–122. doi:10.1080/13614568.2014.983558.

Dudas, R. A., & Crocetti, M. (2013). Pediatric caregiver attitudes toward email communication: Survey in an urban primary care setting. *Journal of Medical Internet Research, 15*(10), 197–204. doi:10.2196/jmir.2738.

Duggan, A. P., & Thompson, T. L. (2011). Patient-provider communication and health outcomes. In T. L. Thompson, R. L. Parrott, & J. Nussbaum (Eds.), *The handbook of health communication* (pp. 414–427). New York: Routledge.

Durant, K. T., McCray, A. T., & Safran, C. (2010). Social network analysis of an online melanoma discussion group. In *Proceedings of the Summit on Translational Bioinformatics* (pp. 6–10). https://www.ncbi.nlm.nih.gov/pmc/articles/PMC3041535/.

Dutta-Bergman, M. J. (2004). Interpersonal communication after 9/11 via telephone and Internet: A theory of channel complementarity. *New Media & Society, 6*(5), 659–673. doi:10.1177/1461444804047086.

Dutta-Bergman, M. J. (2006). Media use theory and Internet use for health care. In M. Murero & R. E. Rice (Eds.), *The Internet and health care* (pp. 83–103). Mahwah, NJ: Lawrence Erlbaum Associates.

Eastin, M. S., & Guinsler, N. M. (2006). Worried and wired: Effects of health anxiety on information-seeking and health care utilization behaviors. *Cyberpsychology & Behavior, 9*(4), 494–498. doi:10.1089/cpb.2006.9.494.

Eastin, M. S., & LaRose, R. (2005). Alt.support: Modeling social support online. *Computers in Human Behavior, 21*, 977–992. doi:10.1017/S0714980811000109.

Egnoto, M. J., Sirianni, J. M., Ortega, C. R., & Stefanone, M. (2014). Death on the digital landscape: A preliminary investigation into the grief process and motivations behind participation in the online memoriam. *Omega, 69*(3), 283–304. doi:10.2190/OM.69.3.d.

Eisenberg, L. (1977). Disease and illness: Distinctions between professional and popular ideas of sickness. *Culture, Medicine and Psychiatry, 1*(1), 9–23. doi:10.1007/BF00114808.

Emanuel, E. J., & Emanuel, L. L. (1992). Four models of the physician-patient relationship. *Journal of the American Medical Association, 267*(16), 2221–2226. doi:10.1001/jama.1992.03480160079038.

Engel, G. (1977). The need for a new medical model: A challenge for biomedicine. *Science, 196*(4286), 129–136. doi:10.1126/science.847460.

Epstein, R. M., Franks, P., Fiscella, K., Shields, G. C., Meldrum, S. C., Kravitz, R. L., & Duberstein, P. R. (2005). Measuring patient-centered communication in patient-physician consultations: Theoretical and practical issues. *Social Science & Medicine, 61*(7), 1516–1528. doi:10.1016/j.socscimed.2005.02.001.

Esquivel, A., Meric-Bernstam, F., & Bernstam, E. V. (2006). Accuracy and self-correction of information received from an internet breast cancer list: Content analysis. *BMJ (Clinical Research Ed.), 332*(7547), 939–942.

Fazeli Dehkordy, S., Carlos, R. C., Hall, K. S., & Dalton, V. K. (2014). Novel data sources for women's health research: Mapping breast screening online information seeking through Google trends. *Academic Radiology, 21*(9), 1172–1176. doi:10.1109/TBME.2011.2132132.

Feng, B., Li, S., & Li, N. (2016). Is a profile worth a thousand words? How online support-seekers profile features may influence the quality of received support messages. *Communication Research, 43*(2), 253–276. doi:10.1177/0093650213510942.

Fergie, G., Hilton, S., & Hunt, K. (2016). Young adults' experiences of seeking online information about diabetes and mental health in the age of social media. *Health Expectations, 19*(6), 1324–1335. doi:10.1111/hex.12430.

Ferguson, R. D., Massimi, M., Crist, E. A., & Moffatt, K. A. (2014). Craving, creating, and constructing comfort: Insights and opportunities for technology in hospice. In *Proceedings of the 17th ACM Conference on Computer Supported Cooperative Work & Social Computing* (pp. 1479–1490). New York, NY: ACM. doi:10.1145/2531602.2531631.

Field, M. J. (1996). *Telemedicine: A guide to assessing telecommunications for health care.* Washington, DC: National Academies Press.

Fife, B. L., & Wright, E. R. (2000). The dimensionality of stigma: A comparison of its impact on the self of persons with HIV/AIDS and cancer. *Journal of Health and Social Behavior, 41*(1), 50–67. doi:10.2307/2676360.

Figueiredo, M. I., Fries, E., & Ingram, K. M. (2004). The role of disclosure patterns and unsupportive social interactions in the well-being of breast cancer patients. *Psycho-Oncology, 13*(2), 96–105. doi:10.1002/pon.717.

Folkman, S., & Lazarus, R. S. (1980). An analysis of coping in a middle-aged community sample. *Journal of Health and Social Behavior, 21*(3), 219–239.

Folkman, S., & Lazarus, R. S. (1985). If it changes it must be a process: Study of emotion and coping during three stages of a college examination. *Journal of Personality and Social Psychology, 48*(1), 150–170. doi:10.1037/0022-3514.48.1.150.

Fox, S. (2011). Peer-to-peer healthcare. *Pew Internet and American Life Project.* Retrieved from http://pewinternet.org/Reports/2011/P2PHealthcare.aspx.

Fox, S., & Duggan, M. (2013). Health online. *Pew Internet and American Life Project.* Retrieved from http://pewinternet.org/Reports/2013/Health-online.aspx.

Fox, S., & Rainie, L. (2000). The online health care revolution: How the web helps Americans take better care of themselves. *Pew Internet and American Life Project.* Retrieved from http://www.pewinternet.org/.

Frank, A. W. (2013). *The wounded storyteller: Body, illness, and ethics.* Chicago, IL: University of Chicago Press.

Frattaroli, J. (2006). Experimental disclosure and its moderators: A meta-analysis. *Psychological Bulletin, 132*(6), 823–865. doi:10.1037/0033-2909.132.6.823.

Fredrickson, B. L. (2001). The role of positive emotions in positive psychology: The broaden-and-build theory of positive emotions. *American Psychologist, 56*(3), 218–226. doi:10.1037/0003-066X.56.3.218.

Freeston, M. H., Rhéaume, J., Letarte, H., Dugas, M. J., & Ladouceur, R. (1994). Why do people worry? *Personality and Individual Differences, 17*(6), 791–802. doi:10.1016/0191-8869(94)90048-5.

Frisina, P. G., Borod, J. C., & Lepore, S. J. (2004). A meta-analysis of the effects of written emotional disclosure on the health outcomes of clinical populations. *Journal of Nervous and Mental Disease, 192*(9), 629–634. doi:10.1097/01.nmd.0000138317. 30764.63.

Fu, K.-W., Wong, P. W. C., & Yip, P. S. F. (2010). What do internet users seek to know about depression from web searches? Descriptive study of 21 million web queries. *Journal of Clinical Psychiatry, 71*(9), 1246–1247. doi:10.4088/JCP.09l05903blu.

Fuoco, M., & Leveridge, M. J. (2015). Early adopters or laggards? Attitudes toward and use of social media among urologists. *BJU International, 115*(3), 491–497. doi:10.1111/bju.12855.

Gage, E. A., & Panagakis, C. (2012). The devil you know: Parents seeking information online for paediatric cancer. *Sociology of Health & Illness, 34*(3), 444–458. doi:10.1111/j.1467-9566.2011.01386.x.

Gao, G. G., McCullough, J. S., Agarwal, R., & Jha, A. K. (2012). A changing landscape of physician quality reporting: Analysis of patients' online ratings of their physicians over a 5-year period. *Journal of Medical Internet Research, 14*(1), e38. doi:10.2196/jmir.2003.

Gaster, B., Knight, C. L., DeWitt, D. E., Sheffield, J. V. L., Assefi, N. P., & Buchwald, D. (2003). Physicians' use of and attitudes toward electronic mail for patient communication. *Journal of General Internal Medicine, 18*(5), 385–389. doi:10.1046/j. 1525-1497.2003.20627.x.

Gavin, J., Rodham, K., & Poyer, H. (2008). The presentation of "pro-anorexia" in online group interactions. *Qualitative Health Research, 18*(3), 325–333. doi:10.1177/ 1049732307311640.

Gerrits, R. S., van der Zanden, R. A. P., Visscher, R. F. M., & Conijn, B. P. (2007). Master your mood online: A preventive chat group intervention for adolescents. *Australian e-Journal for the Advancement of Mental Health, 6*(3), 1–11. doi:10.5172/ jamh.6.3.152.

Getty, E., Cobb, J., Gabeler, M., Nelson, C., Weng, E., & Hancock, J. (2011). I said your name in an empty room: Grieving and continuing bonds on Facebook. In *Proceedings of the SIGCHI Conference on Human Factors in Computing Systems* (pp. 997–1000). New York, NY: ACM. doi:10.1145/1978942.1979091.

Ghaddar, S. F., Valerio, M. A., Garcia, C. M., & Hansen, L. (2012). Adolescent health literacy: The importance of credible sources for online health information. *Journal of School Health, 82*(1), 28–36. doi:10.1111/j.1746-1561.2011.00664.x.

Gibbs, M., Meese, J., Arnold, M., Nansen, B., & Carter, M. (2015). #Funeral and Instagram: Death, social media, and platform vernacular. *Information Communication and Society, 18*(3), 255–268. doi:10.1080/1369118X.2014.987152.

Gibson, J. J. (1977). A theory of affordances. In R. Shaw & R. Bransford (Eds.), *Perceiving, acting, and knowing: Toward an ecological psychology* (pp. 67–82). Hillsdale, NJ: Lawrence Erlbaum Associates.

Gibson, M., & Altena, M. (2014). The digital lives of the dead: YouTube as a practice of cybermourning. In D. M. Dun & S. Dun (Eds.), *A Digital Janus: Looking forward, looking back* (pp. 15–27). Oxford, UK: Inter-Disciplinary Press.

Gimpel, H., Nißen, M., & Gorlitz, R. A. (2013). *Quantifying the quantified self: A study on the motivation of patients to track their own health.* Paper presented at the 34th International Conference on Information Systems, Milan, Italy.

Ginossar, T. (2008). Online participation: A content analysis of differences in utilization of two online cancer communities by men and women, patients and family members. *Health Communication, 23*(1), 1–12. doi:10.1080/10410230701697100.

Goffman, E. (1963). *Stigma: Notes on the management of spoiled identity.* Englewood Cliffs, NJ: Prentice-Hall Inc.

Goodwin, R. D., & Friedman, H. S. (2006). Health status and the five-factor personality traits in a nationally representative sample. *Journal of Health Psychology, 11*(5), 643–654. doi:10.1177/1359105306066610.

Gottlieb, B. H., & Bergen, A. E. (2010). Social support concepts and measures. *Journal of Psychosomatic Research, 69*(5), 511–520. doi:10.1016/j.jpsychores.2009.10.001.

Graham, C., Rouncefield, M., & Satchell, C. (2009). Blogging as "therapy"? Exploring personal technologies for smoking cessation. *Health Informatics Journal, 15*(4), 267–281. doi:10.1177/1460458209345897.

Graham, L., Tse, T., & Keselman, A. (2006). Exploring user navigation during online health information seeking. In *AMIA Annual Symposium Proceedings* (pp. 299-303). https://www.ncbi.nlm.nih.gov/pmc/articles/PMC1839467/.

Granovetter, M. S. (1973). The strength of weak ties. *American Journal of Sociology, 78,* 1360–1380. doi:10.1086/225469.

Gray, S. E., & Coulton, P. (2013). Living with the dead: Emergent post-mortem digital curation and creation practices. In C. Maciel & C. V. Pereira (Eds.), *Digital legacy and interaction* (pp. 31–47). New York: Springer International Publishing.

Green-Hamann, S., Campbell Eichhorn, K., & Sherblom, J. C. (2011). An exploration of why people participate in Second Life social support groups. *Journal of Computer-Mediated Communication, 16*(4), 465–491. doi:10.1111/j.1083-6101.2011.01543.x.

Greene, J. A., Choudhry, N. K., Kilabuk, E., & Shrank, W. H. (2011). Online social networking by patients with diabetes: A qualitative evaluation of communication with Facebook. *Journal of General Internal Medicine, 26*(3), 287–292. doi:10.1007/s11606-010-1526-3.

Greene, K. (2009). An integrated model of health disclosure decision-making. In T. Afifi & W. Afifi (Eds.), *Uncertainty and information regulation in interpersonal contexts: Theories and applications* (pp. 226–253). New York: Routledge.

Gustafson, D. H., McTavish, F. M., Stengle, W., Ballard, D., Hawkins, R., Shaw, B. R., ... & Landucci, G. (2005). Use and impact of ehealth system by low-income women with breast cancer. *Journal of Health Communication, 10,* 195–218. doi:10.1080/10810730500263257.

Haas, S. M., Irr, M. E., Jennings, N. A., & Wagner, L. M. (2011). Communicating thin: A grounded model of online negative enabling support groups in the pro-anorexia movement. *New Media & Society, 13*(1), 40–57. doi:10.1177/1461444810363910.

Haberstroh, S., & Moyer, M. (2012). Exploring an online self-injury support group: Perspectives from group members. *Journal for Specialists in Group Work, 37,* 113–132. doi:10.1080/01933922.2011.646088.

Hadert, A., & Rodham, K. (2008). The invisible reality of arthritis: A qualitative analysis of an online message board. *Musculoskeletal Care, 6*(3), 181–196. doi:10.1002/msc.131.

Hall, A., Bosevski, D., & Larkin, R. (2006). Blogging by the dead. In A. Morch, K. Morgan, T. Bratteteig, G. Ghosh, & D. Svanaes (Eds.), *Proceedings of the 4th Nordic Conference on Human-Computer Interaction* (pp. 425–428). New York, NY: ACM. doi:10.1145/1182475.1182528.

Halpert, A., Dalton, C. B., Palsson, O., Morris, C., Hu, Y., Bangdiwala, S., ... & Drossman, D. (2007). What patients know about irritable bowel syndrome (IBS) and what they would like to know. *American Journal of Gastroenterology, 102*(9), 1972–1982. doi:10.1111/j.1572-0241.2007.01254.x.

Hampton, K., Goulet, L. S., Rainie, L., & Purcell, K. (2011). Social networking sites and our lives. *Pew Internet and American Life Project.* Retrieved from http://www.pewinternet.org.

Han, J. Y., Kim, J. H., Yoon, H. J., Shim, M., McTavish, F. M., & Gustafson, D. H. (2012). Social and psychological determinants of levels of engagement with an online breast cancer support group: Posters, lurkers, and nonusers. *Journal of Health Communication, 17*(3), 356–371. doi:10.1080/10810730.2011.585696.

Han, J. Y., Shaw, B. R., Hawkins, R. P., Pingree, S., McTavish, F., & Gustafson, D. H. (2008). Expressing positive emotions within online support groups by women with breast cancer. *Journal of Health Psychology, 13*(8), 1002–1007.

Hardey, M. (1999). Doctor in the house: The Internet as a source of lay health knowledge and the challenge to expertise. *Sociology of Health & Illness, 21*(6), 820–835.

Hardey, M. (2001). "E-health": The internet and the transformation of patients into consumers and producers of health knowledge. *Information Communication and Society, 4*(3), 388–405. doi:10.1080/13691180110044416.

Hardey, M. (2002). "The story of my illness": Personal accounts of illness on the Internet. *Health, 6*(1), 31–46. doi:10.1177/136345930200600103.

Hartig, J., & Viola, J. (2016). Online grief support communities: Therapeutic benefits of membership. *Omega, 73*(1), 29–41. doi:10.1177/0030222815575698.

Healey, B., Hoek, J., & Edwards, R. (2014). Posting behaviour patterns in an online smoking cessation social network: Implications for intervention design and development. *PLoS One, 9*(9), e106603. doi:10.1371/journal.pone.0106603.

Helgeson, V. S. (1993). Two important distinctions in social support: Kind of support and perceived versus received. *Journal of Applied Social Psychology, 23*(10), 825–845. doi:10.1111/j.1559-1816.1993.tb01008.x.

Herring, S. C., Scheidt, L. A., Wright, E., & Bonus, S. (2005). Weblogs as a bridging genre. *Information Technology & People, 18*(2), 142–171. doi:10.1108/09593840510601513.

High, A. C., Oeldorf-Hirsh, A., & Bellur, S. (2014). Misery rarely gets company: The influence of emotional bandwidth on supportive communication on Facebook. *Computers in Human Behavior, 34*, 79–88. doi:10.1016/j.chb.2014.01.037.

High, A. C., & Solomon, D. H. (2014). Communication channel, sex, and the immediate and longitudinal outcomes of verbal person-centered support. *Communication Monographs, 81*, 439–468. doi:10.1080/03637751.2014.933245.

High, A. C., & Steuber, K. R. (2014). An examination of support (in) adequacy: Types, sources, and consequences of social support among infertile women. *Communication Monographs, 81*, 157–178. doi:10.1080/03637751.2013.878868.

Hill, J. H., Burge, S., Haring, A., & Young, R. A. (2012). Communication technology access, use, and preferences among primary care patients: From the residency research network of Texas (RRNeT). *Journal of the American Board of Family Medicine, 25*(5), 625–634.

Himelboim, I. (2008). Reply distribution in online discussions: A comparative network analysis of political and health newsgroups. *Journal of Computer-Mediated Communication, 14*(1), 156–177. doi:10.1111/j.1083-6101.2008.01435.x.

Hinton, L., Kurinczuk, J. J., & Ziebland, S. (2010). Infertility; isolation and the Internet: A qualitative interview study. *Patient Education and Counseling, 81*(3), 436–441. doi:10.1016/j.pec.2010.09.023.

Hogan, T. P., & Brashers, D. E. (2009). The theory of communication and uncertainty management: Implications from the wider realm of information behavior. In

T. D. Afifi & W. A. Afifi (Eds.), *Uncertainty, information management, and disclosure decisions* (pp. 45–66). New York, NY: Routledge.

Holbrey, S., & Colson, N. S. (2013). A qualitative investigation of the impact of peer to peer online support for women living with polycystic ovary syndrome. *BMC Women's Health, 13.* doi:10.1186/1472-6874-13-51.

Holmstrom, A. J., & Burleson, B. R. (2011). An initial test of a cognitive-emotional theory of esteem support messages. *Communication Research, 38*(3), 326–355. doi:10.1177/0093650210376191.

Holt-Lunstad, J., Smith, T. B., & Layton, J. B. (2010). Social relationships and mortality risk: A meta-analytic review. *PLoS Medicine, 7*(7), e1000316. doi:10.1371/journal.pmed.1000316.

Hou, J., & Shim, M. (2010). The role of provider-patient communication and trust in online sources in Internet use for health-related activities. *Journal of Health Communication, 15,* 186–199. doi:10.1080/10810730.2010.522691.

House, J. S. (1980). *Occupational stress and the mental and physical health of factory workers.* Ann Arbor, MI: Institute for Social Research.

House, J. S., Landis, K. R., & Umberson, D. (1988). Social relationships and health. *Science, 241*(4865), 540–545. doi:10.1126/science.3399889.

Houston, T. K., Cooper, L. A., & Ford, D. E. (2002). Internet support groups for depression: A 1-year prospective cohort study. *American Journal of Psychiatry, 159,* 2062–2068. doi:10.1176/appi.ajp.159.12.2062.

Houston, T. K., Sands, D. Z., Nash, B. R., & Ford, D. E. (2003). Experiences of physicians who frequently use e-mail with patients. *Health Communication, 15*(4), 515–525. doi:10.1207/S15327027HC1504_08.

Høybye, M. T., Johansen, C., & Tjørnhøj-Thomsen, T. (2005). Online interaction: Effects of storytelling in an Internet breast cancer support group. *Psycho-Oncology, 14*(3), 211–220. doi:10.1002/pon.837.

Hoyt, T., & Pasupathi, M. (2008). Blogging about trauma: Linguistic markers of apparent recovery. *E-Journal of Applied Psychology : Clinical and Social Issues, 4*(2), 56–62. doi:10.7790/ejap.v4i2.106.

Hu, Y., & Sundar, S. S. (2010). Effects of online health sources on credibility and behavioral intentions. *Communication Research, 37*(1), 105–132. doi:10.1177/0093650209351512.

Huang, G. C., Unger, J. B., Soto, D., Fujimoto, K., Pentz, M. A., Jordan-Marsh, M., & Valente, T. W. (2014). Peer influences: The impact of online and offline friendship networks on adolescent smoking and alcohol use. *Journal of Adolescent Health, 54*(5), 508–514. doi:10.1016/j.jadohealth.2013.07.001.

Huh, J. (2015). Clinical questions in online health communities: The case of "see your doctor" threads. In *Proceedings of the 18th ACM Conference on Computer Supported Cooperative Work* (pp. 1488–1499). New York, NY: ACM. doi:10.1145/2675133.2675259.

Hume, J., & Bressers, B. (2009). Obituaries online: New connections with the living: And the dead. *Omega, 60*(3), 255–271. doi:10.2190/OM.60.3.d.

Hunter, E. G. (2008). Beyond death: Inheriting the past and giving to the future, transmitting the legacy of one's self. *Omega, 56*(4), 313–329. doi:10.2190/OM.56.4.a.

Hwang, K. O., Ottenbacher, A. J., Lucke, J. F., Etchegaray, J. M., Graham, A. L., & Thomas, E. J. (2011). Measuring social support for weight loss in an Internet weight loss community. *Journal of Health Communication, 16*, 198–211. doi:10.1080/10810730.2010.535106.

Hydén, L. C. (1997). Illness and narrative. *Sociology of Health & Illness, 19*(1), 48–69. doi:10.1111/j.1467-9566.1997.tb00015.x.

Im, E.-O., Chee, W., Liu, Y., Lim, H. J., Guevara, E., Tsai, H.-M., ... & Kim, Y. H. (2007). Characteristics of cancer patients in internet cancer support groups. *Computers, Informatics, Nursing, 25*(6), 334–343.

Introne, J., Semaan, B., & Goggins, S. (2016). A sociotechnical mechanism for online support provision. In *Proceedings of the 2016 CHI Conference on Human Factors in Computing Systems* (pp. 3559–3571). New York, NY: ACM. doi:10.1145/2858036.2858582.

Ireland, M. E., & Pennebaker, J. W. (2010). Language style matching in writing: Synchrony in essays, correspondence, and poetry. *Journal of Personality and Social Psychology, 99*(3), 549–571. doi:10.1037/a0020386.

Irwin, M. D. (2015). Mourning 2.0: Continuing bonds between the living and the dead on Facebook. *Omega, 72*(2), 119–150.

Jackson, D., & Usher, K. (2015). Understanding expressions of public grief: "Mourning sickness," "grief-lite," or something more? *International Journal of Mental Health Nursing, 24*(2), 93–94. doi:10.1111/inm.12127.

Jadhav, A., Andrews, D., Fiksdal, A., Kumbamu, A., McCormick, J. B., Misitano, A., ... & Pathak, J. (2014). Comparative analysis of online health queries originating from personal computers and smart devices on a consumer health information portal. *Journal of Medical Internet Research, 16*(7), e160. doi:10.2196/jmir.3186.

Jain, A., Petty, E. M., Jaber, R. M., Tackett, S., Purkiss, J., Fitzgerald, J., & White, C. (2014). What is appropriate to post on social media? Ratings from students, faculty members and the public. *Medical Education, 48*(2), 157–169. doi:10.1111/medu.12282.

Jamieson, K. H., & Campbell, K. K. (1982). Rhetorical hybrids: Fusions of generic elements. *Quarterly Journal of Speech, 68*(2), 146–157. doi:10.1080/00335638209383600.

Jamison-Powell, S., Briggs, P., Lawson, S., Lineham, C., Windle, K., & Gross, H. (2016). PS I love you: Understanding the impact of posthumous digital messages. In *Proceedings of the CHI Conference on Human Factors in Computing Systems* (pp. 2920–2932). New York, NY: ACM. doi:10.1145/2858036.2858504.

Jensen, J. D., King, A. J., Davis, L. A., & Guntzviller, L. M. (2010). Utilization of Internet technology by low-income adults: The role of health literacy, health numeracy, and computer assistance. *Journal of Aging and Health, 22*(6), 804–826. doi:10.1177/0898264310366161.

Jenssen, B. P., Mitra, N., Shah, A., Wan, F., & Grande, D. (2016). Using digital technology to engage and communicate with patients: A survey of patient attitudes. *Journal of General Internal Medicine, 31*(1), 85–92. doi:10.1007/s11606-015-3517-x.

John, O., Naumann, L., & Soto, C. (2008). Paradigm shift to the integrative big five trait taxonomy: History, measurement, and conceptual issues. In O. John, R. Robbins, & L. Pervin (Eds.), *Handbook of Personality* (pp. 114–156). New York, NY: Guilford.

Johnson, J. D. (1997). *Cancer-related information seeking*. Cresskill, NJ: Hampton Press.

Johnson, J. D., & Case, D. O. (2012). *Health information seeking*. New York, NY: Peter Lang.

Johnson, J. D., & Meischke, H. (1993). A comprehensive model of cancer-related information seeking applied to magazines. *Human Communication Research, 19*(3), 343–367. doi:10.1111/j.1468-2958.1993.tb00305.x.

Jones, L. M., Veinot, T. C. E., Pressler, S. J., Seng, J. S., McCall, A. M., Fernandez, D., & Coleman-Burns, P. W. (2014). Internet health information seeking (IHIS): An integrative review of the literature. *Western Journal of Nursing Research, 36*(10), 1376–1377. doi:10.1177/0193945914540100.

Jones, S. (2004). 404 not found: The Internet and the afterlife. *Omega, 49*(1), 83–88. doi:10.2190/8UUF-GLEG-X6T5-UNJM.

Kaczmarek, L. D., & Krazkowski, D. (2014). MMORPG escapism predicts decreased well-being: Examination of game time, game realism beliefs, and online social support for offline problems. *Cyberpsychology, Behavior, and Social Networking, 17,* 298–302. doi:10.1089/cyber.2013.0595.

Kadry, B., Chu, L. F., Kadry, B., Gammas, D., & Macario, A. (2011). Analysis of 4999 online physician ratings indicates that most patients give physicians a favorable rating. *Journal of Medical Internet Research*, *13*(4), e95. doi:10.3928/01477447 -20090728-04.

Kalichman, S. C., Cherry, C., Cain, D., Weinhardt, L. S., Benotsch, E., Pope, H., & Kalichman, M. (2006). Health information on the Internet and people living with HIV/AIDS: Information evaluation and coping styles. *Health Psychology*, *25*(2), 205– 210. doi:10.1037/0278-6133.25.2.205.

Kanouse, D. E., Schlesinger, M., Shaller, D., Martino, S. C., & Rybowski, L. (2016). How patient comments affect consumers' use of physician performance measures. *Medical Care*, *54*(1), 24–31. doi:10.1097/MLR.0000000000000443.

Kantrowitz-Gordon, I. (2013). Internet confessions of postpartum depression. *Issues in Mental Health Nursing*, *34*(12), 874–882. doi:10.3109/01612840.2013.806618.

Kaplan, A. M., & Haenlein, M. (2010). Users of the world, unite! The challenges and opportunities of social media. *Business Horizons*, *53*(1), 59–68. doi:10.1016/ j.bushor.2009.09.003.

Karras, E., & Rintamaki, L. S. (2012). An examination of online health information seeking by deaf people. *Health Communication*, *27*(2), 194–204. doi:10.1080/ 10410236.2011.575539.

Kayhan, V. O. (2013). Seeking health information on the web: Positive hypothesis testing. *International Journal of Medical Informatics*, *82*(4), 268–275. doi:10.1016/ j.ijmedinf.2012.12.004.

Keating, D. M. (2013). Spirituality and support: A descriptive analysis of online social support for depression. *Journal of Religion and Health*, *52*(3), 1014–1028. doi:10.1007/s10943-012-9577-x.

Keeley, M. P. (2015). End-of-life communication. In C. R. Berger & M. E. Roloff (Eds.), *The international encyclopedia of interpersonal communication*. New York, NY: Wiley-Blackwell; 10.1002/9781118540190.wbeic015.

Keim-Malpass, J., & Steeves, R. H. (2012). Talking with death at a diner: Young women's online narratives of cancer. *Oncology Nursing Forum*, *39*(4), 373–378. doi:10.1188/12.ONF.373-378.

Kern, R., Forman, A. E., & Gil-Egui, G. (2013). RIP: Remain in perpetuity: Facebook memorial pages. *Telematics and Informatics*, *30*(1), 2–10. doi:10.1016/j.tele.2012. 03.002.

Ketteridge, G., Delbridge, H., & Delbridge, L. (2005). How effective is email communication for patients requiring elective surgery? *ANZ Journal of Surgery*, *75*(8), 680–683.

Khoo, K., Bolt, P., Babl, F. E., Jury, S., & Goldman, R. D. (2008). Health information seeking by parents in the Internet age. *Journal of Paediatrics and Child Health, 44*(7–8), 419–423. doi:10.1111/j.1440-1754.2008.01322.x.

Kiesler, S., Siegel, J., & McGuire, T. W. (1984). Social psychological aspects of computer-mediated communication. *American Psychologist, 39,* 1123–1134. doi:10.1037/0003-066X.39.10.1123.

Kim, E., Han, J. Y., Moon, T. J., Shaw, B., Shah, D. V., McTavish, F., & Gustafson, D. H. (2012). The process and effects of supportive message expression and reception in online breast cancer support groups. *Psycho-Oncology, 21,* 531–540. doi:10.1002/pon.1942.

Kim, E., Han, J. Y., Shah, D., Shaw, B., McTavish, F., Gustafson, D. H., & Fan, D. (2011). Predictors of supportive message expression and reception in an interactive cancer communication system. *Journal of Health Communication, 16*(10), 1106–1121. doi:10.1080/10810730.2011.571337.

Kim, E., Hou, J., Han, J. Y., & Himelboim, I. (2016). Predicting retweeting behavior on breast cancer social networks: Network and content characteristics. *Journal of Health Communication, 21*(4), 479–486. doi:10.1080/10810730.2015.1103326.

Kim, H. (2014). Enacted support on social media and subjective well-being. *International Journal of Communication, 8,* 2201–2221.

Kim, H. N., Garfield, C., & Lee, Y. S. (2015). Paternal and maternal information and communication technology usage as their very low birth weight infants transition home from the NICU. *International Journal of Human-Computer Interaction, 31*(1), 44–54. doi:10.1080/10447318.2014.959102.

Kim, J., & Dindia, K. (2011). Online self-disclosure: A review of research. In K. B. Wright & L. M. Webb (Eds.), *Computer-mediated communication in personal relationships* (pp. 156–180). New York, NY: Peter Lang Publishing.

Kim, S. (2009). Content analysis of cancer blog posts. *Journal of the Medical Library Association: JMLA, 97*(4), 260–266. doi:10.3163/1536-5050.97.4.009.

Kim, S. C., Shah, D. V., Namkoong, K., McTavish, F. M., & Gustafson, D. H. (2013). Predictors of online health information seeking among women with breast cancer: The role of social support perception and emotional well-being. *Journal of Computer-Mediated Communication, 18*(2), 98–118. doi:10.1111/jcc4.12002.

Kirschning, S., & von Kardorff, E. (2008). The use of the Internet by women with breast cancer and men with prostate cancer: Results of online research. *Journal of Public Health, 16*(2), 133–143. doi:10.1007/s10389-007-0134-0.

Kivits, J. (2006). Informed patients and the Internet: A mediated context for consultations with health professionals. *Journal of Health Psychology, 11*(2), 269–282. doi:10.1177/1359105306061186.

Klastrup, L. (2015). "I didn't know her, but … ": Parasocial mourning of mediated deaths on Facebook RIP pages. *New Review of Hypermedia and Multimedia, 21*(1–2), 146–164. doi:10.1080/13614568.2014.983564.

Klee, D., Covey, C., & Zhong, L. (2015). Social media beliefs and usage among family medicine residents and practicing family physicians. *Family Medicine, 47*(3), 222–226.

Kleinman, A. (1988). *The illness narratives: Suffering, healing, and the human condition.* New York, NY: Basic Books, Inc.

Ko, H. C., & Kuo, F. Y. (2009). Can blogging enhance subjective well-being through self-disclosure? *Cyberpsychology & Behavior, 12*, 75–79. doi:10.1089/cpb.2008.016.

Kontos, E., Blake, K. D., Chou, W.-Y. S., & Prestin, A. (2014). Predictors of ehealth usage: Insights on the digital divide from the Health Information National Trends Survey 2012. *Journal of Medical Internet Research, 16*(7), e172. doi:10.2196/jmir.3117.

Kozlov, E., & Carpenter, B. D. (2015). "What is palliative care?": Variability in content of palliative care informational web pages. *American Journal of Hospice & Palliative Care, 34*(3), 241–247. doi:10.1177/1049909115615566.

Kraut, R., Kiesler, S., Boneva, B., Cummings, J. N., Helgeson, V., & Crawford, A. M. (2002). Internet paradox revisited. *Journal of Social Issues, 58*(1), 49–74. doi:10.1111/1540-4560.00248.

Krysinska, K., & Andriessen, K. (2010). On-line support and resources for people bereaved through suicide: What is available? *Suicide & Life-Threatening Behavior, 40*(6), 640–650. doi:10.1521/suli.2010.40.6.640.

Krysinska, K., & Andriessen, K. (2015). Online memorialization and grief after suicide: An analysis of suicide memorials on the Internet. *Omega, 71*(1), 19–47. doi:10.1177/0030222814568276.

Krysinska, K., Andriessen, K., & Corveleyn, J. (2014). Religion and spirituality in online suicide bereavement: An analysis of online memorials. *Crisis, 35*(5), 349–356. doi:10.1027/0227-5910/a000270.

Kuehn, B. M. (2013). More than one-third of US individuals use the Internet to self-diagnose. *Journal of the American Medical Association, 309*(8), 756–757. doi:10.1001/jama.2013.629.

Kunkel, A. D., & Dennis, M. R. (2003). Grief consolation in eulogy rhetoric: An integrative framework. *Death Studies, 27*(1), 1–38. doi:10.1080/07481180302872.

LaCoursiere, S. P. (2001). A theory of online social support. *Advances in Nursing Science, 24*(1), 60–77.

Lagoe, C., & Atkin, D. (2015). Health anxiety in the digital age: An exploration of psychological determinants of online health information seeking. *Computers in Human Behavior, 52*, 484–491. doi:10.1016/j.chb.2015.06.003.

Lakey, B., & Cohen, S. (2000). Social support theory and measurement. In S. Cohen, L. Underwood, & B. Gottlieb (Eds.), *Measuring and intervening in social support* (pp. 29–52). New York, NY: Oxford University Press.

Lambert, S. D., & Loiselle, C. G. (2007). Health information-seeking behavior. *Qualitative Health Research, 17*(8), 1006–1019. doi:10.1177/1049732307305199.

Laugesen, J., Hassanein, K., & Yuan, Y. (2015). The impact of Internet health information on patient compliance: A research model and an empirical study. *Journal of Medical Internet Research, 17*(6), e143. doi:10.2196/jmir.4333.

Laurent, M. R., Cremers, S., Verhoef, G., & Dierickx, D. (2012). Internet use for health information among haematology outpatients: A cross-sectional survey. *Informatics for Health & Social Care, 37*(2), 62–73. doi:10.3109/17538157.2011.606481.

Lazarus, R. S. (1966). *Psychological stress and the coping process*. New York, NY: McGraw-Hill.

Lazarus, R. S. (1993). Coping theory and research: Past, present, and future. *Psychosomatic Medicine, 55*(3), 234–247. doi:10.1097/00006842-199305000-00002.

Lazarus, R. S. (2012). Evolution of a model of stress, coping, and discrete emotions. In V. H. Rice (Ed.), *Handbook of stress, coping, and health* (pp. 199–225). Thousand Oaks, CA: Sage.

Lazarus, R. S., & Folkman, S. (1984). *Stress, appraisal, and coping*. New York, NY: Springer Publishing Company, Inc.

Ledbetter, A. M. (2008). Chronemic cues and sex differences in relational e-mail: Perceiving immediacy and supportive message quality. *Social Science Computer Review, 26*(4), 466–482. doi:10.1177/0894439308314812.

Lee, C.-J. (2008). Does the Internet displace health professionals? *Journal of Health Communication, 13*(5), 450–464. doi:10.1080/10810730802198839.

Lee, C.-J., & Chae, J. (2016). An initial look at the associations of a variety of health-related online activities with cancer fatalism. *Health Communication, 31*(11), 1375–1384. doi:10.1080/10410236.2015.1072885.

Lee, J. L., Choudhry, N. K., Wu, A. W., Matlin, O. S., Brennan, T. A., & Shrank, W. H. (2016). Patient use of email, Facebook, and physician websites to communicate with physicians: A national online survey of retail pharmacy users. *Journal of General Internal Medicine, 31*(1), 45–51. doi:10.1007/s11606-015-3374-7.

Lee, K., Hoti, K., Hughes, J. D., & Emmerton, L. (2014). Dr Google and the consumer: A qualitative study exploring the navigational needs and online health information-seeking behaviors of consumers with chronic health conditions. *Journal of Medical Internet Research, 16*(12), e262. doi:10.2196/jmir.3706.

Leggatt-Cook, C., & Chamberlain, K. (2012). Blogging for weight loss: Personal accountability, writing selves, and the weight-loss blogosphere. *Sociology of Health & Illness, 34*(7), 963–977. doi:10.1111/j.1467-9566.2011.01435.x.

Leonard, L. G., & Toller, P. (2012). Speaking ill of the dead: Anonymity and communication about suicide on MyDeathSpace.com. *Communication Studies, 63*(4), 387–404. doi:10.1080/10510974.2011.629274.

Leonardi, P. M., Huysman, M., & Steinfield, C. (2013). Enterprise social media: Definition, history, and prospects for the study of social technologies in organizations. *Journal of Computer-Mediated Communication, 19*(1), 1–19. doi:10.1111/jcc4.12029.

Leong, S. L., Gingrich, D., Lewis, P. R., Mauger, D. T., & George, J. H. (2005). Enhancing doctor-patient communication using email: A pilot study. *Journal of the American Board of Family Practice, 18*(3), 180–188.

Lepore, S. J., Greenberg, M. A., Bruno, M., & Smyth, J. M. (2002). Expressive writing and health: Self-regulation of emotional-related experience, physiology, and behavior. In S. J. Lepore & J. M. Smyth (Eds.), *The writing cure: How expressive writing promotes health and emotional well-being* (pp. 99–117). Washington, DC: American Psychological Association.

Lewallen, A. C., Owen, J. E., Bantum, E. O. C., & Stanton, A. L. (2014). How language affects peer responsiveness in an online cancer support group: Implications for treatment design and facilitation. *Psycho-Oncology, 23*(7), 766–772. doi:10.1002/pon.3477.

Lewandowski, J., Rosenberg, B. D., Parks, M. J., & Siegel, J. T. (2011). The effect of informal social support: Face-to-face versus computer-mediated communication. *Computers in Human Behavior, 27*, 1806–1814. doi:10.1016/j.chb.2011.03.008.

Lewis, N., Gray, S. W., Freres, D. R., & Hornik, R. C. (2009). Examining cross-source engagement with cancer-related information and its impact on doctor-patient relations. *Health Communication, 24*(8), 723–734. doi:10.1080/10410230903264030.

Li, J., Theng, Y.-L., & Foo, S. (2015). Predictors of online health information seeking behavior: Changes between 2002 and 2012. *Health Informatics Journal, 22*, 804–814. doi:10.1177/1460458215595851.

Li, N., Orrange, S., Kravitz, R. L., & Bell, R. A. (2014). Reasons for and predictors of patients' online health information seeking following a medical appointment. *Family Practice, 31*(5), 550–556. doi:10.1093/fampra/cmu034.

Li, S., Feng, B., Chen, M., & Bell, R. A. (2015). Physician review websites: Effects of the proportion and position of negative reviews on readers' willingness to choose the doctor. *Journal of Health Communication, 20*(4), 453–461. doi:10.1080/10810730. 2014.977467.

Liang, T.-P., Ho, Y.-T., Li, Y.-W., & Turban, E. (2011). What drives social commerce: The role of social support and relationship quality. *International Journal of Electronic Commerce, 16*(2), 69–90.

Lieberman, M. (2007). The role of insightful disclosure in outcomes for women in peer-directed breast cancer groups: A replication study. *Psycho-Oncology, 16*(10), 961–964. doi:10.1002/pon.1181.

Lieberman, M. A., & Goldstein, B. A. (2006). Not all negative emotions are equal: The role of emotional expression in online support groups for women with breast cancer. *Psycho-Oncology, 15*, 160–168. doi:10.1002/pon.932.

Lingel, J. (2013). The digital remains: Social media and practices of online grief. *Information Society, 29*(3), 190–195. doi:10.1080/01972243.2013.777311.

Liszka, H. A., Steyer, T. E., & Hueston, W. J. (2006). Virtual medical care: How are our patients using online health information? *Journal of Community Health, 31*(5), 368–378.

Liu, C., & Yu, C. (2013). Can Facebook induce well-being. *Cyberpsychology, Behavior, and Social Networking, 16*, 674–678. doi:10.1089/cyber.2012.0301.

Liu, L. S., Inkpen, K. M., & Pratt, W. (2015). "I'm not like my friends": Understanding how children with a chronic illness use technology to maintain normalcy. In *Proceedings of the 18th ACM Conference on Computer Supported Cooperative Work & Social Computing* (pp. 1527–1539). New York, NY: ACM. doi:10.1145/2675133. 2675201.

Liu, X., & LaRose, R. (2008). Does using the Internet make people more satisfied with their lives? The effects of the Internet on college students' school life satisfaction. *Cyberpsychology & Behavior, 11*, 310–319. doi:10.1089/cpb.2007.0040.

Locasto, M. E., Massimi, M., & DePasquale, P. J. (2011). Security and privacy considerations in digital death. In *Proceedings of the 2011 Workshop on New Security Paradigms* (pp. 1–10). New York, NY: ACM. doi:10.1145/2073276.2073278.

Longman, H., O'Connor, E., & Obst, P. (2009). The effect of social support derived from World of Warcraft on negative psychological symptoms. *Cyberpsychology & Behavior, 12*, 563–566. doi:10.1089/cpb.2009.001.

Lowney, A., & O'Brien, T. (2012). The landscape of blogging in palliative care. *Palliative Medicine, 26*(6), 858–859. doi:10.1177/0269216311432900.

Lyons, E. J., Mehl, M. R., & Pennebaker, J. W. (2006). Pro-anorexics and recovering anorexics differ in their linguistic internet self-presentation. *Journal of Psychosomatic Research, 60*(3), 253–256. doi:10.1016/j.jpsychores.2005.07.017.

Lyons, R. F., Sullivan, M. J. L., Ritvo, P. G., & Coyne, J. C. (1995). *Relationships in chronic illness and disability*. Thousand Oaks, CA: Sage.

Ma, X., Chen, G., & Xiao, J. (2010). *Analysis of an online health social network*. Paper presented at the 1st ACM International Health Informatics Symposium, Arlington, VA.

MacGeorge, E. L., Feng, B., & Burleson, B. (2011). Supportive communication. In M. L. Knapp & J. A. Daly (Eds.), *Handbook of interpersonal communication* (pp. 317–354). Thousand Oaks, CA: Sage.

MacGeorge, E. L., Feng, B., Butler, G. L., & Budarz, S. K. (2004). Understanding advice in supportive interactions: Beyond the facework and message evaluation paradigm. *Human Communication Research, 30*(1), 42–70. doi:10.1093/hcr/30.1.42.

Malik, S. H., & Coulson, N. S. (2008). Computer-mediated infertility support groups: An exploratory study of online experiences. *Patient Education and Counseling, 73*, 105–113. doi:10.1016/j.pec.2008.05.024.

Maloney, E. K., D'Agostino, T. A., Heerdt, A., Dickler, M., Li, Y., Ostroff, J. S., & Bylund, C. L. (2015). Sources and types of online information that breast cancer patients read and discuss with their doctors. *Palliative & Supportive Care, 13*(2), 107–114. doi:10.1017/S1478951513000862.

Mankoff, J., Kuksenok, K., Kiesler, S., Rode, J. A., & Waldman, K. (2011). Competing online viewpoints and models of chronic illness. In *Proceedings of the SIGCHI Conference on Human Factors in Computing Systems* (pp. 589–598). New York, NY: ACM. doi:10.1145/1978942.1979027.

Marcus, M. A., Westra, H. A., Eastwood, J. D., & Barnes, K. L. (2012). What are young adults saying about mental health? An analysis of Internet blogs. *Journal of Medical Internet Research, 14*(1), e17. doi:10.2196/jmir.1868.

Markle, G. L., Attell, B. K., & Treiber, L. A. (2015). Dual, yet dueling illnesses: Multiple chronic illness experience at midlife. *Qualitative Health Research, 25*(9), 1271–1282. doi:10.1177/1049732314559948.

Markus, M. L., & Silver, M. S. (2008). A foundation for the study of IT effects: A new look at DeSanctis and Poole's concepts of structural features and spirit. *Journal of the Association for Information Systems, 9*(10/11), 609–632.

Marwick, A., & Ellison, N. (2012). "There isn't wifi in heaven!" Negotiating visibility on Facebook memorial pages. *Journal of Broadcasting & Electronic Media, 56*(3), 378–400. doi:10.1080/08838151.2012.705197.

Massimi, M. (2013). Exploring remembrance and social support behavior in an online bereavement support group. In *Proceedings of the 2013 Conference on Computer Supported Cooperative Work* (pp. 1169–1180). New York, NY: ACM. doi:10.1145/2441776.2441908.

Maudlin, J., Keene, J., & Kobb, R. (2006). A road map for the last journey: Home telehealth for holistic end-of-life care. *American Journal of Hospice and Palliative Medicine, 23*(5), 399–403. doi:10.1177/1049909106290807.

McCallig, D. (2014). Facebook after death: An evolving policy in a social network. *International Journal of Law and Information Technology, 22*(2), 107–140. doi:10.1093/ijlit/eat012.

McCosker, A., & Darcy, R. (2013). Living with cancer: Affective labour, self-expression and the utility of blogs. *Information Communication and Society, 16*(8), 1266–1285. doi:10.1080/1369118X.2012.758303.

McDaniel, B. T., Coyne, S. M., & Holmes, E. K. (2012). New mothers and media use: Associations between blogging, social networking, and maternal well-being. *Maternal and Child Health Journal, 16*, 1509–1517. doi:10.1007/s10995-011-0918-2.

McGowan, B. S., Wasko, M., Vartabedian, B. S., Miller, R. S., Freiherr, D. D., & Abdol-rasulnia, M. (2012). Understanding the factors that influence the adoption and meaningful use of social media by physicians to share medical information. *Journal of Medical Internet Research, 14*(5), 210–220. doi:10.2196/jmir.2138.

McKay, H. G., Glasgow, R. E., Feil, E. G., Boles, S. M., & Barrera, M., Jr. (2002). Internet-based diabetes self-management and support: Initial outcomes from the diabetes network project. *Rehabilitation Psychology, 47*(1), 31–48. doi:10.1037/0090-5550.47.1.31.

McKenna, K. Y. A., & Bargh, J. A. (1998). Coming out in the age of the Internet: Identity "demarginalization" through virtual group participation. *Journal of Personality and Social Psychology, 75*(3), 681–694. doi:10.1037/0022-3514.75.3.681.

McKenna, K. Y. A., & Bargh, J. A. (2000). Plan 9 from cyberspace: The implications of the Internet for personality and social psychology. *Personality and Social Psychology Review, 4*(1), 57–75. doi:10.1207/S15327957PSPR0401_6.

McKinley, C. J., & Ruppel, E. K. (2014). Exploring how perceived threat and self-efficacy contribute to college students' use and perceptions of online mental health resources. *Computers in Human Behavior, 34*, 101–109. doi:10.1016/j.chb.2014.01.038.

McPherson, A. C., Gofine, M. L., & Stinson, J. (2014). Seeing is believing? A mixed-methods study exploring the quality and perceived trustworthiness of online information about chronic conditions aimed at children and young people. *Health Communication, 29*(5), 473–482. doi:10.1080/10410236.2013.768325.

MedlinePlus. (2015). MedlinePlus guide to healthy web surfing. Retrieved from http://medlineplus.gov/healthywebsurfing.html.

Medlock, S., Eslami, S., Askari, M., Sent, D., de Rooij, S. E., & Abu-Hanna, A. (2013). The consequences of seniors seeking health information using the internet and other sources. *Studies in Health Technology and Informatics, 192*, 457–460. doi:10. 3233/978-1-61499-289-9-457.

Meese, J., Nansen, B., Kohn, T., Arnold, M., & Gibbs, M. (2015). Posthumous personhood and the affordances of digital media. *Mortality, 20*(4), 408–420. doi:10.1080/ 13576275.2015.1083724.

Menachemi, N., Prickett, C. T., & Brooks, R. G. (2011). The use of physician-patient email: A follow-up examination of adoption and best-practice adherence 2005–2008. *Journal of Medical Internet Research, 13*(1), e23. doi:10.2196/jmir.1578.

Meng, J. (2016). Your health buddies matter: Preferential selection and social influence on weight management in an online health social network. *Health Communication, 31*(12), 1460–1471. doi:10.1080/10410236.2015.1079760.

Meng, J., Chung, M., & Cox, J. (2016). Linking network structure to support messages: Effects of brokerage and closure on received social support. *Journal of Communication, 66*(6), 982–1006. doi:10.1111/jcom.12268.

Merolli, M., Gray, K., & Martin-Sanchez, F. (2014). Therapeutic affordances of social media: Emergent themes from a global online survey of people with chronic pain. *Journal of Medical Internet Research, 16*(12), e284. doi:10.2196/jmir.3494.

Meylakhs, P., Rykov, Y., Koltsova, O., & Koltsov, S. (2014). An AIDS-denialist online community on a Russian social networking service: Patterns of interactions with newcomers and rhetorical strategies of persuasion. *Journal of Medical Internet Research, 16*(11), e261. doi:10.2196/jmir.3338.

Miller, E. A., & Pole, A. (2010). Diagnosis blog: Checking up on health blogs in the blogosphere. *American Journal of Public Health, 100*(8), 1514–1519. doi:10.2105/ AJPH.2009.175125.

Mirivel, J. C., & Thombre, A. (2010). Surviving online: An analysis of how burn survivors recover from life crises. *Southern Communication Journal, 75*(3), 232–254. doi:10.1080/10417940903377151.

Mo, P. K., & Coulson, N. S. (2013). Online support group use and psychological health for individuals living with HIV/AIDS. *Patient Education and Counseling, 93*, 426–432. doi:10.1016/j.pec.2013.04.004.

Mo, P. K. H., & Coulson, N. S. (2010). Empowering processes in online support groups among people living with HIV/AIDS: A comparative analysis of "lurkers" and "posters." *Computers in Human Behavior, 26*(5), 1183–1193. doi:10.1016/j.chb. 2010.03.028.

Moncur, W., Bikker, J., Kasket, E., & Troyer, J. (2012). From death to final disposition: Roles of technology in the post-mortem interval. In *Proceedings of the SIGCHI Conference on Human Factors in Computing Systems* (pp. 531–540). New York, NY: ACM. doi:10.1145/2207676.2207750.

Moyer, C. A., Stern, D. T., Dobias, K. S., Cox, D. T., & Katz, S. J. (2002). Bridging the electronic divide: Patient and provider perspectives on e-mail communication in primary care. *American Journal of Managed Care, 8*(5), 427–433.

Mulveen, R., & Hepworth, J. (2006). An interpretative phenomenological analysis of participation in a pro-anorexia Internet site and its relationship with disordered eating. *Journal of Health Psychology, 11*(2), 283–296. doi:10.1177/1359105306061187.

Munir, F., Leka, S., & Griffiths, A. (2005). Dealing with self-management of chronic illness at work: Predictors for self-disclosure. *Social Science & Medicine, 60*(6), 1397–1407. doi:10.1016/j.socscimed.2004.07.012.

Muse, K., McManus, F., Leung, C., Meghreblian, B., & Williams, J. M. G. (2012). Cyberchondriasis: Fact or fiction? A preliminary examination of the relationship between health anxiety and searching for health information on the Internet. *Journal of Anxiety Disorders, 26*(1), 189–196. doi:10.1016/j.janxdis.2011.11.005.

Myneni, S., Fujimoto, K., Cobb, N., & Cohen, T. (2015). Content-driven analysis of an online community for smoking cessation: Integration of qualitative techniques, automated text analysis, and affiliation networks. *American Journal of Public Health, 105*(6), 1206–1212. doi:10.2105/AJPH.2014.302464.

Nagel, D., & Anthony, K. (2009). Writing therapy using new technologies: The art of blogging. *Journal of Poetry Therapy, 22*(1), 41–45. doi:10.1080/08893670802708001.

Naslund, J. A., Grande, S. W., Aschbrenner, K. A., & Elwyn, G. (2014). Naturally occurring peer support through social media: The experiences of individuals with severe mental illness using YouTube. *PLoS One, 9*(10), e110171. doi:10.1371/journal.pone.0110171.

National Cancer Institute. (2003). *Health Information National Trends Survey* [dataset].

National Cancer Institute. (2005). *Health Information National Trends Survey* [dataset].

National Cancer Institute. (2011). *Health Information National Trends Survey* [dataset].

National Cancer Institute. (2013). *Health Information National Trends Survey* [dataset].

National Cancer Institute. (2015). *Health Information National Trends Survey* [dataset].

National Telecommunication and Information Agency. (2004). *A nation online: Entering the broadband age*. Retrieved from https://www.ntia.doc.gov.

Neelapala, P., Duvvi, S. K., Kumar, G., & Kumar, B. N. (2008). Do gynaecology out-patients use the Internet to seek health information? A questionnaire survey. *Journal of Evaluation in Clinical Practice, 14*(2), 300–304. doi:10.1111/j.1365-2753.2007.00854.x.

Newnham, G. M., Burns, W. I., Snyder, R. D., Dowling, A. J., Ranieri, N. F., Gray, E. L., et al. (2006). Information from the Internet: Attitudes of Australian oncology patients. *Internal Medicine Journal, 36*(11), 718–723. doi:10.1111/j.1445-5994. 2006.01212.

Nguyen, M., Bin, Y. S., & Campbell, A. (2012). Comparing online and offline self-disclosure: A systematic review. *Cyberpsychology, Behavior, and Social Networking, 15*(2), 103–111. doi:10.1089/cyber.2011.0277.

Nolen-Hoeksema, S., McBride, A., & Larson, J. (1997). Rumination and psychological distress among bereaved partners. *Journal of Personality and Social Psychology, 72*(4), 855–862. doi:10.1037/0022-3514.72.4.855.

Norman, D. A. (1999). Affordance, conventions, and design. *Interaction, 6*(3), 38–43.

Norr, A. M., Albanese, B. J., Oglesby, M. E., Allan, N. P., & Schmidt, N. B. (2015). Anxiety sensitivity and intolerance of uncertainty as potential risk factors for cyberchondria. *Journal of Affective Disorders, 174*, 64–69. doi:10.1016/j.jad.2014.11.023.

North, R. L., & Rothenberg, K. H. (1993). Partner notification and the threat of domestic violence against women with HIV infection. *New England Journal of Medicine, 329*(16), 1194–1196. doi:10.1056/nejm199310143291612.

Nwosu, A. C., Debattista, M., Rooney, C., & Mason, S. (2015). Social media and palliative medicine: A retrospective 2-year analysis of global Twitter data to evaluate the use of technology to communicate about issues at the end of life. *BMJ Supportive & Palliative Care, 5*(2), 207–212. doi:10.1136/bmjspcare-2014-000701.

Odom, W., Harper, R., Sellen, A., Kirk, D., & Banks, R. (2010). Passing on & putting to rest: Understanding bereavement in the context of interactive technologies. In *Proceedings of the SIGCHI Conference on Human Factors in Computing Systems* (pp. 1831–1840). New York, NY: ACM. doi:10.1145/1753326.1753601.

Oh, H. J., Lauckner, C., Boehmer, J., Fewins-Bliss, R., & Li, K. (2013). Facebooking for health: An examination into the solicitation and effects of health-related social support on social networking sites. *Computers in Human Behavior, 29*, 2072–2080. doi:10.1016/j.chb.2013.04.017.

Oh, H. J., & Lee, B. (2012). The effect of computer-mediated social support in online communities on patient empowerment and doctor-patient interaction. *Health Communication, 27*, 30–41. doi:10.1080/10410236.2011.567449.

Oh, H. J., Ozkaya, E., & LaRose, R. (2014). How does online social networking enhance life satisfaction? The relationships among online supportive interaction, affect, perceived social support, sense of community, and life satisfaction. *Computers in Human Behavior, 30*, 69–78. doi:10.1016/j.chb.2013.07.053.

Oh, Y. S., & Cho, Y. (2015). Examining the relationships between resources and online health information seeking among patients with chronic diseases and healthy people. *Social Work in Health Care, 54*(2), 83–100. doi:10.1080/00981389. 2014.987940.

Oh, Y. S., & Song, N. K. (2017). Investigating relationships between health-related problems and online health information seeking. *Computers, Informatics, Nursing, 35*(1), 29–35. doi:10.1097/CIN.0000000000000234.

Oliver, D. R. P., Demiris, G., Day, M., Courtney, K. L., & Porock, D. (2006). Telehospice support for elder caregivers of hospice patients: Two case studies. *Journal of Palliative Medicine, 9*(2), 264–267. doi:10.1089/jpm.2006.9.264.

Orlikowski, W. J., & Yates, J. (1994). Genre repertoire: The structuring of communicative practices in organizations. *Administrative Science Quarterly, 39*(4), 541–574. doi:10.2307/2393771.

Ostherr, K., Killoran, P., Shegog, R., & Bruera, E. (2016). Death in the digital age: A systematic review of information and communication technologies in end-of-life care. *Journal of Palliative Medicine, 19*(4), 408–420. doi:10.1089/jpm.2015.0341.

Owen, J. E., Curran, M., Bantum, E. O. C., & Hanneman, R. (2016). Characterizing social networks and communication channels in a web-based peer support intervention. *Cyberpsychology, Behavior, and Social Networking, 19*(6), 388–396. doi:10.1089/cyber.2015.0359.

Owen, J. E., Klapow, J. C., Roth, D. L., Shuster, J. L., Jr., Bellis, J., Meredith, R., & Tucker, D. C. (2005). Randomized pilot of a self-guided internet coping group for women with early-stage breast cancer. *Annals of Behavioral Medicine, 30*(1), 54–64. doi:10.1207/s15324796abm3001_7.

Owen, J. E., Klapow, J. C., Roth, D. L., & Tucker, D. C. (2004). Use of the Internet for information and support: Disclosure among persons with breast and prostate cancer. *Journal of Behavioral Medicine, 27*(5), 491–505. doi:10.1023/B:JOBM.0000047612.81370.f7.

Palotti, J., Hanbury, A., Müller, H., & Kahn, C. E. (2016). How users search and what they search for in the medical domain. *Information Retrieval Journal, 19*(1), 189–224. doi:10.1007/s10791-015-9269-8.

Pang, C. E., Neustaedter, C., Riecke, B. E., Oduor, E., & Hillman, S. (2013). Technology preferences and routines for sharing health information during the treatment of a chronic illness. In *Proceedings of the SIGCHI Conference on Human Factors in Computing Systems* (pp. 1759–1768). New York, NY: ACM. doi:10.1145/2470654.2466232.

Paolino, L., Genser, L., Fritsch, S., De' Angelis, N., Azoulay, D., & Lazzati, A. (2015). The web-surfing bariatric patient: The role of the internet in the decision-making process. *Obesity Surgery, 25*(4), 738–743. doi:10.1007/s11695-015-1578-x.

Park, C. L. (2010). Making sense of the meaning literature: An integrative review of meaning making and its effects on adjustment to stressful life events. *Psychological Bulletin, 136*(2), 257–301. doi:10.1037/a0018301.

Park, C. L., & Folkman, S. (1997). Meaning in the context of stress and coping. *Review of General Psychology, 1*(2), 115–144. doi:10.1037/1089-2680.1.2.115.

Patt, M. R., Houston, T. K., Jenckes, M. W., Sands, D. Z., & Ford, D. E. (2003). Doctors who are using e-mail with their patients: A qualitative exploration. *Journal of Medical Internet Research, 5*(2), e9.

Pennebaker, J. W. (1997). *Opening up: The healing power of expressing emotions.* New York, NY: Guilford Press.

Pennebaker, J. W., & Chung, C. K. (2007). Expressive writing, emotional upheavals, and health. In H. S. Friedman & R. C. Silver (Eds.), *Foundations of health psychology* (pp. 263–284). New York, NY: Oxford University Press.

Pennebaker, J. W., Chung, C. K., Ireland, M., Gonzales, A., & Booth, R. J. (2007). *The development and psychometric properties of LIWC2007.* Austin, TX: LIWC.net.

Pennebaker, J. W., Mayne, T. J., & Francis, M. E. (1997). Linguistic predictors of adaptive bereavement. *Journal of Personality and Social Psychology, 72*(4), 863–871. doi:10.1037/0022-3514.72.4.863.

Percheski, C., & Hargittai, E. (2011). Health information-seeking in the digital age. *Journal of American College Health, 59*(5), 379–386. doi:10.1080/07448481.2010.513406.

Pereira, J., Bruera, E., Macmillan, K., & Kavanagh, S. (2000). Palliative cancer patients and their families on the Internet: Motivation and impact. *Journal of Palliative Care, 16*(4), 13–19.

Pereira, J., Bruera, E., & Quan, H. (2001). Palliative care on the net: An online survey of health care professionals. *Journal of Palliative Care, 17*(1), 41–45.

Perez, S. L., Paterniti, D. A., Wilson, M., Bell, R. A., Chan, M. S., Villareal, C. C., ... & Kravitz, R. L. (2015). Characterizing the processes for navigating Internet health information using real-time observations: A mixed-methods approach. *Journal of Medical Internet Research, 17*(7), e173. doi:10.2196/jmir.3945.

Perrin, A., & Duggan, M. (2015). Americans' Internet access: 2000–2015. *Pew Internet and American Life Project.* Retrieved from http://www.pewinternet.org.

Pew Internet and American Life Project. (2012). *Health Tracking Survey 2012* [dataset].

Pizziferri, L., Kittler, A., Volk, L. A., Hobbs, J., Jagannath, Y., & Wald, J. S., & Bates, D. W. (2003). Physicians' perceptions toward electronic communication with patients. In *AMIA Annual Symposium Proceedings* (pp. 972–972). https://www.ncbi.nlm.nih.gov/pmc/articles/PMC1480248/.

Politi, M. C., & Street, R. L. (2011). The importance of communication in collaborative decision making: Facilitating shared mind and the management of uncertainty.

Journal of Evaluation in Clinical Practice, 17(4), 579–584. doi:10.1111/j.1365-2753. 2010.01549.x.

Possemato, K., Ouimette, P., & Geller, P. A. (2010). Internet-based expressive writing for kidney transplant recipients: Effects on posttraumatic stress and quality of life. *Traumatology, 16*(1), 49–54. doi:10.1177/1534765609347545.

Powell, J., & Clarke, A. (2006). Internet information-seeking in mental health: Population survey. *British Journal of Psychiatry, 189*(3), 273–277. doi:10.1192/bjp.bp. 105.017319.

Prates, R. O., Rosson, M. B., & de Souza, C. S. (2015). Making decisions about digital legacy with Google's inactive account manager. In J. Abascal, S. Barbosa, M. Fetter, T. Gross, P. Palanque, & M. Winckler (Eds.), *Human-computer interaction—INTERACT 2015* (pp. 201–209). New York, NY: Springer.

Prestin, A., Vieux, S. N., & Chou, W.-Y. S. (2015). Is online health activity alive and well or flatlining? Findings from 10 years of the Health Information National Trends Survey. *Journal of Health Communication, 20*(7), 790–798. doi:10.1080/10810730. 2015.1018590.

Prybutok, G., & Ryan, S. (2015). Social media: The key to health information access for 18- to 30-year-old college students. *Computers, Informatics, Nursing. CIN, 33*(4), 132–141. doi:10.1097/CIN.0000000000000147.

Qiu, B., Zhao, K., Mitra, P., Wu, D., Caragea, C., & Yen, J., & Portier, K. (2011). *Get online support, feel better: Sentiment analysis and dynamics in an online cancer survivor community.* Paper presented at the 2011 IEEE Third International Conference on Privacy, Security, Risk and Trust, Boston, MA.

Radin, P. (2006). "To me, it's my life": Medical communication, trust, and activism in cyberspace. *Social Science & Medicine, 62*(3), 591–601.

Rainie, L., & Fox, S. (2000). The online health care revolution. *Pew Internet and American Life Project.* Retrieved from http://www.pewinternet.org.

Rains, S. A. (2007a). The anonymity effect: The influence of anonymity on perceptions of sources and information on health websites. *Journal of Applied Communication Research, 35*(2), 197–214. doi:10.1080/00909880701262666.

Rains, S. A. (2007b). Perceptions of traditional information sources and use of the World Wide Web to seek health information: Findings from the Health Information National Trends Survey. *Journal of Health Communication, 12*(7), 667–680. doi:10. 1080/10810730701619992.

Rains, S. A. (2008). Seeking health information in the information age: The role of Internet self-efficacy. *Western Journal of Communication, 72*(1), 1–18. doi:10.1080/ 10570310701827612.

Rains, S. A. (2014a). Health information seeking and the World Wide Web: An uncertainty management perspective. *Journal of Health Communication, 19*(11), 1296–1307. doi:10.1080/10810730.2013.872731.

Rains, S. A. (2014b). The implications of stigma and anonymity for self-disclosure in health blogs. *Health Communication, 29*(1), 23–31. doi:10.1080/10410236.2012. 714861.

Rains, S. A. (2016). Language style matching as a predictor of perceived social support in computer-mediated interaction among individuals coping with illness. *Communication Research, 43*(5), 694–712. doi:10.1177/0093650214565920.

Rains, S. A., Brunner, S. R., Akers, C., Pavlich, C. A., & Goktas, S. (2017). Computer-mediated communication (CMC) and social support: Testing the effects of using CMC on support outcomes. *Journal of Social and Personal Relationships, 34*(8), 1186–1205. doi:10.1177/0265407516670533.

Rains, S. A., Brunner, S. R., Akers, C., Pavlich, C. A., & Tsetsi, E. (2016). The implications of computer-mediated communication (CMC) for social support message processing and outcomes: When and why are the effects of support messages strengthened during CMC? *Human Communication Research, 42*(4), 553–576. doi:10.1111/hcre.12087.

Rains, S. A., & Karmikel, C. D. (2009). Health information-seeking and perceptions of website credibility: Examining web-use orientation, message characteristics, and structural features of websites. *Computers in Human Behavior, 25*(2), 544–553. doi:10.1016/j.chb.2008.11.005.

Rains, S. A., & Keating, D. M. (2011). The social dimension of blogging about health: Health blogging, social support, and well-being. *Communication Monographs, 78*, 511–534. doi:10.1080/03637751.2011.618142.

Rains, S. A., & Keating, D. M. (2015). Health blogging: An examination of the outcomes associated with making public, written disclosures about health. *Communication Research, 42*(1), 107–133. doi:10.1177/0093650212458952.

Rains, S. A., Peterson, E. B., & Wright, K. B. (2015). Communicating social support in computer-mediated contexts: A meta-analytic review of content analyses examining support messages shared online among individuals coping with illness. *Communication Monographs, 82*(4), 403–430. doi:10.1080/03637751.2015.1019530.

Rains, S. A., & Ruppel, E. K. (2016). Channel complementarity theory and the health information-seeking process. *Communication Research, 43*(2), 232–252. doi:10.1177/0093650213510939.

Rains, S. A., & Tukachinsky, R. (2015). An examination of the relationships among uncertainty, appraisal, and information-seeking behavior proposed in uncertainty management theory. *Health Communication, 30*(4), 339–349. doi:10.1080/10410236. 2013.858285.

Rains, S. A., & Wright, K. B. (2016). Social support and computer-mediated communication: A state-of-the-art review and agenda for future research. In E. Cohen (Ed.), *Communication yearbook* (pp. 175–212). New York, NY: Routledge.

Rains, S. A., & Young, V. J. (2009). A meta-analysis of research on formal computer-mediated support groups: Examining group characteristics and health outcomes. *Human Communication Research, 35,* 309–336. doi:10.1111/j.1468-2958.2009.01353.x.

Renahy, E., Parizot, I., & Chauvin, P. (2008). Health information seeking on the Internet: A double divide? Results from a representative survey in the Paris metropolitan area, France, 2005–2006. *BMC Public Health, 8,* 69. doi:10.1186/ 1471-2458-8-69.

Ressler, P. K., Bradshaw, Y. S., Gualtieri, L., & Chui, K. K. H. (2012). Communicating the experience of chronic pain and illness through blogging. *Journal of Medical Internet Research, 14*(5), e143. doi:10.2196/jmir.2002.

Rice, R. E. (2006). Influences, usage, and outcomes of Internet health information searching: Multivariate results from the Pew surveys. *International Journal of Medical Informatics, 75*(1), 8–28. doi:10.1016/j.ijmedinf.2005.07.032.

Rider, T., Malik, M., & Chevassut, T. (2014). Haematology patients and the Internet: The use of on-line health information and the impact on the patient-doctor relationship. *Patient Education and Counseling, 97*(2), 223–238. doi:10.1016/j. pec.2014.06.018.

Riggs, N. A. (2014). Following Bud blogging at the end-of-life. *Qualitative Inquiry, 20*(3), 376–384. doi:10.1177/1077800413505539.

Roberts, K. J. (1999). Patient empowerment in the United States: A critical commentary. *Health Expectations, 2*(2), 82–92.

Roberts, P. (2012). "2 people like this": Mourning according to format. *Bereavement Care, 31*(2), 55–61. doi:10.1080/02682621.2012.710492.

Roberts, P., & Vidal, L. A. (2000). Perpetual care in cyberspace: A portrait of memorials on the web. *Omega, 40*(4), 521–545. doi:10.2190/3BPT-UYJR-192R-U969.

Robinson, J. D., Turner, J. W., Levine, B., & Tian, Y. (2011). Expanding the walls of the health care encounter: Support and outcomes for patients online. *Health Communication, 26*(2), 125–134. doi:10.1080/10410236.2010.541990.

Rodham, K., McCabe, C., & Blake, D. (2009). Seeking support: An interpretative phenomenological analysis of an Internet message board for people with complex regional pain syndrome. *Psychology & Health, 24*(6), 619–634. doi:10.1080/ 08870440802563245.

Rodriquez, J. (2013). Narrating dementia: Self and community in an online forum. *Qualitative Health Research, 23*(9), 1215–1227. doi:10.1177/1049732313501725.

Rosen, N. O., Knäuper, B., & Sammut, J. (2007). Do individual differences in intolerance of uncertainty affect health monitoring? *Psychology & Health, 22*(4), 413–430. doi:10.1080/14768320600941038.

Rosen, P., & Kwoh, C. K. (2007). Patient-physician e-mail: An opportunity to transform pediatric health care delivery. *Pediatrics, 120*(4), 701–706. doi:10.1542/peds.2007-1094.

Rosenquist, J. N. (2011). Lessons from social network analyses for behavioral medicine. *Current Opinion in Psychiatry, 24*(2), 139–143. doi:10.1097/YCO.0b013e3283438061.

Rossetto, K. R., Lannutti, P. J., & Strauman, E. C. (2015). Death on Facebook: Examining the roles of social media communication for the bereaved. *Journal of Social and Personal Relationships, 32*(7), 974–994. doi:10.1177/0265407514555272.

Roter, D. L., & Hall, J. A. (2006). *Doctors talking with patients/patients talking with doctors*. Westport, CT: Praeger.

Roter, D. L., Larson, S., Sands, D. Z., Ford, D. E., & Houston, T. (2008). Can e-mail messages between patients and physicians be patient-centered? *Health Communication, 23*(1), 80–86. doi:10.1080/10410230701807295.

Roter, D. L., & McNeilis, K. S. (2003). The nature of the therapeutic relationship and the assessment of its discourse in routine medical visits. In T. L. Thompson, A. M. Dorsey, K. I. Miller, & R. Parrott (Eds.), *Handbook of health communication* (pp. 121–140). Mahwah, NJ: Lawrence Erlbaum Associates.

Royer, A. (1998). *Life with chronic illness: Social and psychological dimensions*. Westport, CT: Praeger.

Ruiz, I. S., García, G. P., & Riquelme, I. (2014). E-mail communication in pain practice: The importance of being earnest. *Saudi Journal of Anaesthesia, 8*(3), 364–367. doi:10.4103/1658-354X.136434.

Ruppel, E. K., Gross, C., Stoll, A., Peck, B. S., Allen, M., & Kim, S.-Y. (2017). Reflecting on connecting: Meta-analysis of differences between computer-mediated and face-to-face self-disclosure. *Journal of Computer-Mediated Communication, 22*(1), 18–34. doi:10.1111/jcc4.12179.

Ruppel, E. K., & McKinley, C. J. (2015). Social support and social anxiety in use and perceptions of online mental health resources: Exploring social compensation and enhancement. *Cyberpsychology, Behavior, and Social Networking, 18*(8), 462–467. doi:10.1089/cyber.2014.0652.

Ruppel, E. K., & Rains, S. A. (2012). Information sources and the health information-seeking process: An application and extension of channel complementarity theory. *Communication Monographs, 79*(3), 385–405. doi:10.1080/03637751.2012.697627.

Ruthven, I. (2012). Grieving online: The use of search engines in times of grief and bereavement. In *Proceedings of the 4th Information Interaction in Context Symposium* (pp. 120–128). New York, NY: ACM. doi:10.1145/2362724.2362747.

Sabee, C. M., Bylund, C. L., Weber, J. G., & Sonet, E. (2012). The association of patients' primary interaction goals with attributions for their doctors' responses in conversations about online health research. *Journal of Applied Communication Research, 40*(3), 271–288. doi:10.1080/00909882.2012.679671.

Samal, L., Saha, S., Chander, G., Korthuis, P. T., Sharma, R. K., Sharp, V., ... & Beach, M. C. (2011). Internet health information seeking behavior and antiretroviral adherence in persons living with HIV/AIDS. *AIDS Patient Care and STDs, 25*(7), 445–449. doi:10.1089/apc.2011.0027.

Sanford, A. A. (2010). "I can air my feelings instead of eating them": Blogging as social support for the morbidly obese. *Communication Studies, 61*(5), 567–584. doi:10.1080/10510974.2010.514676.

Santana, S., Lausen, B., Bujnowska-Fedak, M., Chronaki, C., Kummervold, P. E., Rasmussen, J., & Sorensen, T. (2010). Online communication between doctors and patients in Europe: Status and perspectives. *Journal of Medical Internet Research, 12*(2), e20. doi:10.2196/jmir.1281.

Sassenberg, K., & Greving, H. (2016). Internet searching about disease elicits a positive perception of own health when severity of illness is high: A longitudinal questionnaire study. *Journal of Medical Internet Research, 18*(3), e56. doi:10.2196/jmir.5140.

Scambler, G. (2009). Health-related stigma. *Sociology of Health & Illness, 31*(3), 441–455. doi:10.1111/j.1467-9566.2009.01161.x.

Scanfeld, D., Scanfeld, V., & Larson, E. L. (2010). Dissemination of health information through social networks: Twitter and antibiotics. *American Journal of Infection Control, 38*(3), 182–188. doi:10.1016/j.ajic.2009.11.004.

Schulz, P. J., Zufferey, M. C., & Hartung, U. (2011). First check the Internet, then see the doctor: How many patients do it, and who are they? *Studies in Communication Sciences, 11*(2), 99–131.

Sciamanna, C. N., Clark, M. A., Diaz, J. A., & Newton, S. (2003). Filling the gaps in physician communication. The role of the Internet among primary care patients. *International Journal of Medical Informatics, 72*(1–3), 1–8.

Seçkin, G. (2013). Satisfaction with health status among cyber patients: Testing a mediation model of electronic coping support. *Behaviour & Information Technology*, *32*, 91–101. doi:10.1080/0144929X.2011.603359.

Segal, J., Sacopulos, M., Sheets, V., Thurston, I., Brooks, K., & Puccia, R. (2012). Online doctor reviews: Do they track surgeon volume, a proxy for quality of care? *Journal of Medical Internet Research*, *14*(2), e50. doi:10.2196/jmir.2005.

Segrin, C. (2001). *Interpersonal processes in psychological problems.* New York, NY: Guilford Press.

Selby, P., van Mierlo, T., Voci, S. C., Parent, D., & Cunningham, J. A. (2010). Online social and professional support for smokers trying to quit: An exploration of first time posts from 2562 members. *Journal of Medical Internet Research*, *12*(3), 92–102. doi:10.2196/jmir.1340.

Sharf, B. F. (1997). Communicating breast cancer on-line: Support and empowerment on the Internet. *Women & Health*, *26*(1), 65–84. doi:10.1300/J013v26n01_05.

Sharf, B. F., & Vanderford, M. L. (2003). Illness narratives and the social construction of health. In T. L. Thompson, A. M. Dorsey, K. I. Miller, & R. Parrott (Eds.), *Handbook of health communication* (pp. 9–34). Mahwah, NJ: Lawrence Erlbaum Associates.

Shaw, B. R., Hawkins, R., McTavish, F., Pingree, S., & Gustafson, D. H. (2006). Effects of insightful disclosure within computer mediated support groups on women with breast cancer. *Health Communication*, *19*(2), 133–142. doi:10.1207/s15327027hc1902_5.

Shcherbakova, N., & Shepherd, M. (2014). Community pharmacists, internet and social media: An empirical investigation. *Research in Social & Administrative Pharmacy*, *10*(6), e75–e85. doi:10.1016/j.sapharm.2013.11.007.

Sheese, B. E., Brown, E. L., & Graziano, W. G. (2004). Emotional expression in cyberspace: Searching for moderators of the Pennebaker disclosure effect via e-mail. *Health Psychology*, *23*(5), 457–464. doi:10.1037/0278-6133.23.5.457.

Shieh, C., Mays, R., McDaniel, A., & Yu, J. (2009). Health literacy and its association with the use of information sources and with barriers to information seeking in clinic-based pregnant women. *Health Care for Women International*, *30*(11), 971–988. doi:10.1080/07399330903052152.

Shigaki, C. L., Smarr, K. L., Gong, Y., Donovan-Hanson, K., Siva, C., Johnson, R. A., ... & Musser, D. R. (2008). Social interactions in an online self-management program for rheumatoid arthritis. *Chronic Illness*, *4*(4), 239–246. doi:10.1177/1742395308097862.

Shim, M., Cappella, J. N., & Han, J. Y. (2011). How does insightful and emotional disclosure bring potential health benefits? Study based on online support groups for women with breast cancer. *Journal of Communication, 61*(3), 432–454. doi:10.1111/ j.1460-2466.2011.01555.x.

Shim, M., Kelly, B., & Hornik, R. (2006). Cancer information scanning and seeking behavior is associated with knowledge, lifestyle choices, and screening. *Journal of Health Communication, 11*(Suppl1), 157–172. doi:10.1080/10810730600637475.

Silver, M. P. (2015). Patient perspectives on online health information and communication with doctors: A qualitative study of patients 50 years old and over. *Journal of Medical Internet Research, 17*(1), e19. doi:10.2196/jmir.3588.

Singer, P. A., Martin, D. K., & Kelner, M. (1999). Quality end-of-life care: Patients' perspectives. *Journal of the American Medical Association, 281*(2), 163–168. doi:10. 1001/jama.281.2.163.

Sittig, D. F. (2003). Results of a content analysis of electronic messages (email) sent between patients and their physicians. *BMC Medical Informatics and Decision Making, 3*, 11.

Sittig, D. F., King, S., & Hazlehurst, B. L. (2001). A survey of patient-provider e-mail communication: What do patients think? *International Journal of Medical Informatics, 61*(1), 71–80.

Skinner, E. A., Edge, K., Altman, J., & Sherwood, H. (2003). Searching for the structure of coping: A review and critique of category systems for classifying ways of coping. *Psychological Bulletin, 129*(2), 216–269. doi:10.1037/0033-2909.129.2.216.

Smith, K. P., & Christakis, N. A. (2008). Social networks and health. *Annual Review of Sociology, 34*(1), 405–429. doi:10.1146/annurev.soc.34.040507.134601.

Smith, R. A. (2007). Language of the lost: An explication of stigma communication. *Communication Theory, 17*(4), 462–485. doi:10.1111/j.1468-2885.2007.00307.x.

Smyth, J. M. (1998). Written emotional expression: Effect sizes, outcome types, and moderating variables. *Journal of Consulting and Clinical Psychology, 66*(1), 174–184. doi:10.1037/0022-006X.66.1.174.

Sommerhalder, K., Abraham, A., Zufferey, M. C., Barth, J., & Abel, T. (2009). Internet information and medical consultations: Experiences from patients' and physicians' perspectives. *Patient Education and Counseling, 77*(2), 266–271. doi:10.1016/j.pec. 2009.03.028.

Song, F. W., West, J. E., Lundy, L., & Dahmen, N. S. (2012). Women, pregnancy, and health information online: The making of informed patients and ideal mothers. *Gender & Society, 26*(5), 773–798. doi:10.1177/0891243212446336.

Song, H., Omori, K., Kim, J., Tenzek, K. E., Hawkins, J. M., Lin, W.-Y., … & Jung, J. Y. (2016). Trusting social media as a source of health information: Online surveys comparing the United States, Korea, and Hong Kong. *Journal of Medical Internet Research, 18*(3), e25. doi:10.2196/jmir.4193.

Sontag, S. (1977). *Illness as metaphor.* New York, NY: Farrar, Straus and Giroux.

Spielberg, A. R. (1998). On call and online: Sociohistorical, legal, and ethical implications of e-mail for the patient-physician relationship. *Journal of the American Medical Association, 280*(15), 1353–1359. doi:10.1001/jama.280.15.1353.

Spink, A., Yang, Y., Jansen, J., Nykanen, P., Lorence, D. P., Ozmutlu, S., & Ozmutlu, H. C. (2004). A study of medical and health queries to web search engines. *Health Information and Libraries Journal, 21*(1), 44–51. doi:10.1111/j.1471-1842.2004.00481.x.

Spottswood, E. L., Walther, J. B., Holmstrom, A. R., & Ellison, N. E. (2013). Person-centered emotional support and gender attributions in computer-mediated communication. *Human Communication Research, 39*, 295–316. doi:10.1111/hcre.12006.

Stanton, A. L., Danoff-Burg, S., Cameron, C. L., Bishop, M., Collins, C. A., Kirk, S. B., ... & Twillman, R. (2000). Emotionally expressive coping predicts psychological and physical adjustment to breast cancer. *Journal of Consulting and Clinical Psychology, 68*(5), 875–882. doi:10.1037/0022-006X.68.5.875.

Stanton, A. L., Danoff-Burg, S., Cameron, C. L., & Ellis, A. P. (1994). Coping through emotional approach: Problems of conceptualizaton and confounding. *Journal of Personality and Social Psychology, 66*(2), 350–362. doi:10.1037/0022-3514.66.2.350.

Stanton, A. L., Thompson, E. H., Crespi, C. M., Link, J. S., & Waisman, J. R. (2013). Project connect online: Randomized trial of an internet-based program to chronicle the cancer experience and facilitate communication. *Journal of Clinical Oncology, 31*(27), 3411–3417. doi:10.1200/JCO.2012.46.9015.

Stearns, M., Nambiar, S., Nikolaev, A., Semenov, A., & McIntosh, S. (2014). Towards evaluating and enhancing the reach of online health forums for smoking cessation. *Network Modeling and Analysis in Health Informatics and Bioinformatics, 3*(69), 1–23. doi:10.1007/s13721-014-0069-7.

Stewart, M., Brown, J. B., Donner, A., McWhinney, I. R., Oates, J., Weston, W. W., & Jordan, J. (2000). The impact of patient-centered care on outcomes. *Journal of Family Practice, 49*(9), 796–804.

Street, R. L., Jr., Makoul, G., Arora, N. K., & Epstein, R. M. (2009). How does communication heal? Pathways linking clinician-patient communication to health outcomes. *Patient Education and Counseling, 74*(3), 295–301. doi:10.1016/j.pec.2008.11.015.

Stroebe, M., & Schut, H. (1999). The dual process model of coping with bereavement: Rationale and description. *Death Studies, 23*(3), 197–224. doi:10.1080/074811899201046.

Stroebe, M., & Schut, H. (2010). The dual process model of coping with bereavement: A decade on. *Omega, 61*(4), 273–289. doi:10.2190/OM.61.4.b.

Stroebe, M. S., & Schut, H. (2001). Models of coping with bereavement: A review. In M. S. Stroebe, R. O. Hansson, W. Stroebe, & H. Schut (Eds.), *Handbook of bereavement research* (pp. 375–403). Washington, DC: American Psychological Association.

Suler, J. (2004). The online disinhibition effect. *Cyberpsychology & Behavior, 7*(3), 321–326. doi:10.1089/1094931041291295.

Suls, J., & Rothman, A. (2004). Evolution of the biopsychosocial model: Prospects and challenges for health psychology. *Health Psychology, 23*(2), 119–125. doi:10. 1037/0278-6133.23.2.119.

Sundar, S. S. (2008). The MAIN model: A heuristic approach to understanding technology effects on credibility. In A. J. Flanagin & M. Metzger (Eds.), *Digital media, youth, and credibility* (pp. 73–100). Cambridge, MA: The MIT Press.

Sundar, S. S., Edwards, H. H., Hu, Y., & Stavrositu, C. (2007). Blogging for better health: Putting the "public" back in public health. In M. Tremayne (Ed.), *Blogging, citizenship, and the future of media* (pp. 83–102). New York, NY: Routledge.

Swartwood, R. M., Veach, P. M., Kuhne, J., Lee, H. K., & Ji, K. (2011). Surviving grief: An analysis of the exchange of hope in online grief communities. *Omega, 63*(2), 161–181. doi:10.2190/OM.63.2.d.

Synnot, A. J., Hill, S. J., Garner, K. A., Summers, M. P., Filippini, G., Osborne, R. H., … & Mosconi, P. (2014). Online health information seeking: How people with multiple sclerosis find, assess and integrate treatment information to manage their health. *Health Expectations, 19,* 727–737. doi:10.1111/hex.12253.

Tan, L. (2008). Psychotherapy 2.0: Myspace blogging as self-therapy. *American Journal of Psychotherapy, 62*(2), 143–163.

Tanis, M. (2008a). Health-related online forums: What's the big attraction? *Journal of Health Communication, 13,* 698–714. doi:10.1080/10810730802415316.

Tanis, M. (2008b). What makes the Internet a place to seek social support? In E. A. Konijn, S. Utz, M. Tanis, & S. B. Barnes (Eds.), *Mediated interpersonal communication* (pp. 290–308). New York, NY: Routledge.

Tanis, M., Hartmann, T., & te Poel, F. (2016). Online health anxiety and consultation satisfaction: A quantitative exploratory study on their relations. *Patient Education and Counseling, 99*(7), 1227–1232. doi:10.1016/j.pec.2016.01.021.

Thackeray, R., Crookston, B. T., & West, J. H. (2013). Correlates of health-related social media use among adults. *Journal of Medical Internet Research, 15*(1), 190–201. doi:10.2196/jmir.2297.

Thoits, P. A. (2011). Mechanisms linking social ties and support to physical and mental health. *Journal of Health and Social Behavior, 52*(2), 145–161. doi:10.1177/0022146510395592.

Thomas, L., & Briggs, P. (2014). An older adult perspective on digital legacy. In *Proceedings of the 8th Nordic Conference on Human-Computer Interaction* (pp. 237–246). New York, NY: ACM. doi:10.1145/2639189.2639485.

Thomas, L. J., Scharp, K. M., & Paxman, C. G. (2014). Stories of postpartum depression: Exploring health constructs and help-seeking in mothers' talk. *Women & Health, 54*(4), 373–387. doi:10.1080/03630242.2014.896442.

Thomson, M. D., Siminoff, L. A., & Longo, D. R. (2012). Internet use for prediagnosis symptom appraisal by colorectal cancer patients. *Health Education & Behavior, 39*(5), 583–588.

Tian, Y., & Robinson, J. D. (2008a). Incidental health information use and media complementarity: A comparison of senior and non-senior cancer patients. *Patient Education and Counseling, 71*(3), 340–344. doi:10.1016/j.pec.2008.02.006.

Tian, Y., & Robinson, J. D. (2008b). Media use and health information seeking: An empirical test of complementarity theory. *Health Communication, 23*(2), 184–190. doi:10.1080/10410230801968260.

Tong, S. T., Heinemann-LaFave, D., Jeon, J., Kolodziej-Smith, R., & Warshay, N. (2013). The use of pro-ana blogs for online social support. *Eating Disorders, 21*(5), 408–422. doi:10.1080/10640266.2013.827538.

Townsend, A., Leese, J., Adam, P., McDonald, M., Li, L. C., Kerr, S., & Backman, C. L. (2015). eHealth, participatory medicine, and ethical care: A focus group study of patients' and health care providers' use of health-related Internet information. *Journal of Medical Internet Research, 17*(6), e155. doi:10.2196/jmir.3792.

Trehan, S. K., DeFrancesco, C. J., Nguyen, J. T., Charalel, R. A., & Daluiski, A. (2016). Online patient ratings of hand surgeons. *Journal of Hand Surgery, 41*(1), 98–103. doi:10.1016/j.jhsa.2015.10.006.

Tsuya, A., Sugawara, Y., Tanaka, A., & Narimatsu, H. (2014). Do cancer patients tweet? Examining the Twitter use of cancer patients in Japan. *Journal of Medical Internet Research, 16*(5), e137. doi:10.2196/jmir.3298.

Turner, J. W., Grube, J. A., & Meyers, J. (2001). Developing an optimal match within online communities: An exploration of CMC support communities and traditional support. *Journal of Communication, 51*, 231–251. doi:10.1111/j.1460-2466.2001.tb02879.x.

Turner, J. W., Robinson, J. D., Tian, Y., Neustadtl, A., Angelus, P., Russell, M., ... & Levine, B. (2013). Can messages make a difference? The association between e-mail messages and health outcomes in diabetes patients. *Human Communication Research, 39*(2), 252–268. doi:10.1111/j.1468-2958.2012.01437.x.

Turner-McGrievy, G. M., & Tate, D. F. (2013). Weight loss social support in 140 characters or less: Use of an online social network in a remotely delivered weight loss intervention. *Translational Behavioral Medicine, 3*(3), 287–294. doi:10.1007/s13142-012-0183-y.

Tustin, N. (2010). The role of patient satisfaction in online health information seeking. *Journal of Health Communication, 15*(1), 3–17. doi:10.1080/10810730903465491.

Uchino, B. N. (2009). Understanding the links between social support and physical health: A life-span perspective with emphasis on the separability of perceived and received support. *Perspectives on Psychological Science, 4*(3), 236–255. doi:10.1111/j.1745-6924.2009.01122.x.

Urbanoski, K., van Mierlo, T., & Cunningham, J. (2017). Investigating patterns of participation in an online support group for problem drinking: A social network analysis. *International Journal of Behavioral Medicine, 24*(5), 703–712. doi:10.1007/s12529-016-9591-6.

Usher, W. (2011). A health website recommendation from Gold Coast general practitioners to their patients: A mixed method approach. *Health Education Journal, 70*(2), 117–130.

van der Houwen, K., Stroebe, M., Schut, H., Stroebe, W., & van den Bout, J. (2010). Online mutual support in bereavement: An empirical examination. *Computers in Human Behavior, 26*(6), 1519–1525. doi:10.1016/j.chb.2010.05.019.

van Ingen, E., & Wright, K. B. (2016). Predictors of mobilizing online coping versus offline coping resources after negative life events. *Computers in Human Behavior, 59*, 431–439. doi:10.1016/j.chb.2016.02.048.

van Mierlo, T. (2014). The 1% rule in four digital health social networks: An observational study. *Journal of Medical Internet Research, 16*(2), e33. doi:10.2196/jmir.2966.

van Mierlo, T., Hyatt, D., & Ching, A. T. (2015). Mapping power law distributions in digital health social networks: Methods, interpretations, and practical implications. *Journal of Medical Internet Research, 17*(6), e160. doi:10.2196/jmir.4297.

Virji, A., Yarnall, K. S. H., Krause, K. M., Pollak, K. I., Scannell, M. A., Gradison, M., & Ostbye, T. (2006). Use of email in a family practice setting: Opportunities and challenges in patient- and physician-initiated communication. *BMC Medicine, 4*, 18.

Vlahovic, T. A., Wang, Y.-C., Kraut, R. E., & Levine, J. M. (2014). Support matching and satisfaction in an online breast cancer support community. In *Proceedings of the*

SIGCHI Conference on Human Factors in Computing Systems (pp. 1625–1634). New York, NY: ACM. doi:10.1145/2556288.2557108.

Walter, T., Hourizi, R., Moncur, W., & Pitsillides, S. (2011). Does the internet change how we die and mourn? Overview and analysis. *Omega, 64*(4), 275–302. doi:10.2190/OM.64.4.a.

Walther, J. B. (1996). Computer-mediated communication: Impersonal, interpersonal, and hyperpersonal interaction. *Communication Research, 23*, 1–43. doi:10.1177/009365096023001001.

Walther, J. B., & Boyd, S. (2002). Attraction to computer-mediated social support. In C. A. Lin & D. Atkin (Eds.), *Communication technology and society: Audience adoption and uses* (pp. 153–188). Cresskill, NJ: Hampton Press.

Walther, J. B., & Parks, M. R. (2002). Cues filtered out, cues filtered in: Computer-mediated communication and relationships. In M. L. Knapp & J. A. Daly (Eds.), *Handbook of interpersonal communication* (pp. 529–563). Thousand Oaks, CA: Sage.

Wandel, T. L. (2009). Online empathy: Communicating via Facebook to bereaved college students. *Journal of New Communications Research, 4*(2), 42–53.

Wang, Y.-C., Kraut, R., & Levine, J. M. (2012). To stay or leave? The relationship of emotional and informational support to commitment in online health support groups. In *Proceedings of the Conference on Computer Supported Cooperative Work* (pp. 833–842). New York, NY: ACM. doi:10.1145/2145204.2145329.

Wang, Y.-C., Kraut, R. E., & Levine, J. M. (2015). Eliciting and receiving online support: Using computer-aided content analysis to examine the dynamics of online social support. *Journal of Medical Internet Research, 17*(4), e99. doi:10.2196/jmir.3558.

Welbourne, J. L., Blanchard, A. L., & Wadsworth, M. B. (2013). Motivations in virtual health communities and their relationship to community, connectedness and stress. *Computers in Human Behavior, 29*(1), 129–139. doi:10.1016/j.chb.2012.07.024.

Wen, K. Y., McTavish, F., Kreps, G., Wise, M., & Gustafson, D. (2011). From diagnosis to death: A case study of coping with breast cancer as seen through online discussion group messages. *Journal of Computer-Mediated Communication, 16*(2), 331–361. doi:10.1111/j.1083-6101.2011.01542.x.

Westerlund, M., Hadlaczky, G., & Wasserman, D. (2012). The representation of suicide on the Internet: Implications for clinicians. *Journal of Medical Internet Research, 14*(5), 321–328. doi:10.2196/jmir.1979.

Wethington, E., Glanz, K., & Schwartz, M. D. (2015). Stress, coping, and health behavior. In B. K. Rimer & K. V. Viswanath (Eds.), *Health behavior: Theory, research, and practice* (pp. 223–242). San Francisco, CA: Jossey-Bass.

Wethington, E., & Kessler, R. C. (1986). Perceived support, received support, and adjustment to stressful life events. *Journal of Health and Social Behavior, 27*(1), 78–89. doi:10.2307/2136504.

White, C. B., Moyer, C. A., Stern, D. T., & Katz, S. J. (2004). A content analysis of e-mail communication between patients and their providers: Patients get the message. *Journal of the American Medical Informatics Association, 11*(4), 260–267.

White, R. W., & Horvitz, E. (2014). From health search to healthcare: Explorations of intention and utilization via query logs and user surveys. *Journal of the American Medical Informatics Association, 21*(1), 49–55. doi:10.1136/amiajnl-2012-001473.

Whitten, P., Doolittle, G., & Mackert, M. (2004). Telehospice in Michigan: Use and patient acceptance. *American Journal of Hospice & Palliative Medicine, 21*(3), 191–195. doi:10.1177/104990910402100307.

Whitten, P., Doolittle, G., & Mackert, M. (2005). Providers' acceptance of telehospice. *Journal of Palliative Medicine, 8*(4), 730–735. doi:10.1089/jpm.2005.8.730.

Whitten, P., Doolittle, G., Mackert, M., & Rush, T. (2003). Telehospice carries end-of-life care over the lines. *Nursing Management, 34*(11), 36–39.

Whitten, P., Holtz, B., Meyer, E., & Nazione, S. (2009). Telehospice: Reasons for slow adoption in home hospice care. *Journal of Telemedicine and Telecare, 15*(4), 187–190. doi:10.1258/jtt.2009.080911.

Williams, A. L., & Merten, M. J. (2009). Adolescents' online social networking following the death of a peer. *Journal of Adolescent Research, 24*(1), 67–90. doi:10.1177/0743558408328440.

Williams, J. P., & Goh, Y. X. (2015). Notes on the existential and interactional dimensions of authenticity: A symbolic interactionist study of breast cancer internet forums. *M/C Journal, 18*(1). Retrieved from http://www.journal.media-culture.org.au/index.php/mcjournal/article/view/951.

Williams, P. G., O'Brien, C. D., & Colder, C. R. (2004). The effects of neuroticism and extraversion on self-assessed health and health-relevant cognition. *Personality and Individual Differences, 37*(1), 83–94. doi:10.1016/j.paid.2003.08.001.

Wills, T. A., & Ainette, M. C. (2012). Social networks and social support. In A. Baum, T. A. Revenson, & J. Singer (Eds.), *Handbook of health psychology* (pp. 465–492). New York, NY: Psychology Press.

Wills, T. A., & Shinar, O. (2000). Measuring perceived and received social support. In S. Cohen, L. G. Underwood, & B. H. Gottlieb (Eds.), *Social support measurement and intervention: A guide for health and social scientists* (pp. 86–135). New York, NY: Oxford University Press.

Wittenberg-Lyles, E., Oliver, D. P., Demiris, G., & Baldwin, P. (2010). The ACTive intervention in hospice interdisciplinary team meetings: Exploring family caregiver and hospice team communication. *Journal of Computer-Mediated Communication, 15*(3), 465–481.

Wittenberg-Lyles, E., Washington, K., Oliver, D. P., Shaunfield, S., Gage, L. A., Mooney, M., & Lewis, A. (2015). "It is the 'starting over' part that is so hard": Using an online group to support hospice bereavement. *Palliative & Supportive Care, 13*(2), 351–357. doi:10.1017/S1478951513001235.

Wolf, M., Theis, F., & Kordy, H. (2013). Language use in eating disorder blogs: Psychological implications of social online activity. *Journal of Language and Social Psychology, 32*(2), 212–226. doi:10.1177/0261927X12474278.

Wright, K. B. (1999). Computer-mediated support groups: An examination of relationships among social support, perceived stress, and coping strategies. *Communication Quarterly, 47*, 402–414. doi:10.1080/01463379909385570.

Wright, K. B. (2000). Social support satisfaction, on-line communication apprehension, and perceived life stress within computer-mediated support groups. *Communication Research Reports, 17*, 139–147. doi:10.1080/08824090009388760.

Wright, K. B., & Bell, S. B. (2003). Health-related support groups on the Internet: Linking empirical findings to social support and computer-mediated communication theory. *Journal of Health Psychology, 8*(1), 39–54. doi:10.1177/135910530300800 1429.

Wright, K. B., & Miller, C. H. (2010). A measure of weak tie/strong tie support network preference. *Communication Monographs, 77*, 502–520. doi:10.1080/03637751. 2010.502538.

Wright, K. B., & Rains, S. A. (2013). Weak-tie support network preference, stigma, and health outcomes in computer-mediated support groups. *Journal of Applied Communication Research, 41*, 309–324. doi:10.1080/00909882.2013.792435.

Wright, K. B., Rains, S., & Banas, J. (2010). Weak-tie support network preference and perceived life stress among participants in health-related, computer-mediated support groups. *Journal of Computer-Mediated Communication, 15*, 606–624. doi:10. 1111/j.1083-6101.2009.01505.x.

Wright, K. B., Rosenberg, J., Egbert, N., Ploeger, N., Bernard, D. R., & King, S. (2013). Communication competence, social support, and depression among college students: A model of Facebook and face-to-face support network influence. *Journal of Health Communication, 18*, 41–57. doi:10.1080/10810730.2012.688250.

Wright, N. (2014). Death and the Internet: The implications of the digital afterlife. *First Monday, 19*(6). doi:10.5210/fm.v19i6.4998.

Xu, R., & Zhang, Q. (2016). Understanding online health groups for depression: Social network and linguistic perspectives. *Journal of Medical Internet Research*, *18*(3), e63. doi:10.2196/jmir.5042.

Xu, W. W., Chiu, I. H., Chen, Y., & Mukherjee, T. (2015). Twitter hashtags for health: Applying network and content analyses to understand the health knowledge sharing in a Twitter-based community of practice. *Quality & Quantity*, *49*(4), 1361–1380. doi:10.1007/s11135-014-0051-6.

Yao, T., Zheng, Q., & Fan, X. (2015). The impact of online social support on patients' quality of life and the moderating role of social exclusion. *Journal of Service Research*, *18*(3), 369–383. doi:10.1177/1094670515583271.

Ye, J., Rust, G., Fry-Johnson, Y., & Strothers, H. (2010). E-mail in patient-provider communication: A systematic review. *Patient Education and Counseling*, *80*(2), 266–273. doi:10.1016/j.pec.2009.09.038.

Yeshua-Katz, D., & Martins, N. (2013). Communicating stigma: The pro-ana paradox. *Health Communication*, *28*(5), 499–508. doi:10.1080/10410236.2012.699889.

Yi, J., & Zahn, M. P. (2010). Internet use among Chinese-American breast cancer survivors. *International Quarterly of Community Health Education*, *31*(4), 359–368. doi:10.2190/IQ.31.4.d.

Yli-Uotila, T., Rantanen, A., & Suominen, T. (2014). Online social support received by patients with cancer. *Computers, Informatics, Nursing*, *32*, 118–126. doi:10.1097/CIN.0000000000000028.

Yoo, W., Namkoong, K., Choi, M., Shah, D. V., Tsang, S., Hong, Y., et al. (2014). Giving and receiving emotional support online: Communication competence as a moderator of psychosocial benefits for women with breast cancer. *Computers in Human Behavior*, *30*, 13–22. doi:10.1016/j.chb.2013.07.024.

Young, C. (2013). Community management that works: How to build and sustain a thriving online health community. *Journal of Medical Internet Research*, *15*(6), e119. doi:10.2196/jmir.2501.

Zhang, M., & Yang, C. C. (2015). Using content and network analysis to understand the social support exchange patterns and user behaviors of an online smoking cessation intervention program. *Journal of the Association for Information Science and Technology*, *66*(3), 564–575. doi:10.1002/asi.23189.

Zhang, S., Kang, T., Qiu, L., Zhang, W., Yu, Y., & Elhadad, N. (2017). Cataloguing treatments discussed and used in online Autism communities. In *Proceedings of the International World-Wide Web Conference* (pp. 123–131). doi:10.1145/3038912.3052661

Zhao, K., Wang, X., Cha, S., Cohn, A. M., Papandonatos, G. D., Amato, M. S., … & Graham, A. L. (2016). A multirelational social network analysis of an online health community for smoking cessation. *Journal of Medical Internet Research, 18*(8), e233. doi:10.2196/jmir.5985.

Zhou, Y. Y., Kanter, M. H., Wang, J. J., & Garrido, T. (2010). Improved quality at Kaiser Permanente through e-mail between physicians and patients. *Health Affairs, 29*(7), 1370–1375. doi:10.1377/hlthaff.2010.0048.

Ziebland, S., & Wyke, S. (2012). Health and illness in a connected world: How might sharing experiences on the internet affect people's health? *Milbank Quarterly, 90*(2), 219–249. doi:10.1111/j.1468-0009.2012.00662.x.

Zundel, K. M. (1996). Telemedicine: History, applications, and impact on librarianship. *Bulletin of the Medical Library Association, 84*(1), 71–79.

Index